Anatomy Student's Color-In Handbook

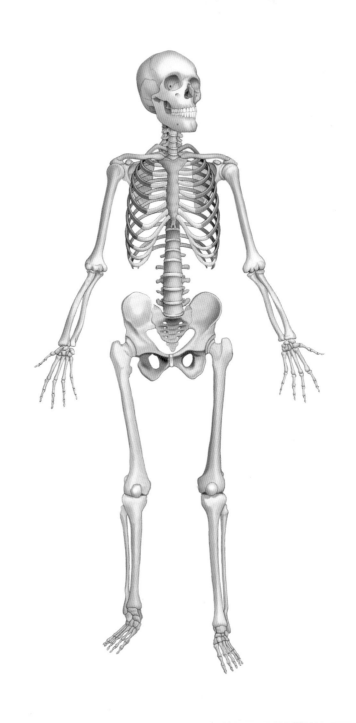

Anatomy Student's Color-In Handbook

VOLUME ONE:

Anatomy Overview • Cells and Tissues
Skeletal System • Joints

Professor Ken Ashwell, BMedSc, MBBS, PhD

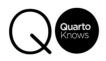

Quarto is the authority on a wide range of topics.

Quarto educates, entertains and enriches the lives of
our readers—enthusiasts and lovers of hands-on living.

www.QuartoKnows.com

First published in 2017 by
Global Book Publishing Pty Ltd
Part of The Quarto Group
Level One, Ovest House,
58 West Street, Brighton, BN1 2RA, UK

ISBN: 978-0-85762-512-0

A Global Book

Printed and bound in China

Conceived, designed and produced by Global Book Publishing

Consultant Editor: Professor Ken Ashwell, BMedSc, MBBS, PhD

Designer: Angela English

Project Editor: Kathleen Steeden

Illustrations:
Joanna Culley, BA(Hons) RMIP, MMAA, IMI (Medical-Artist.com), Mike Gorman,
Thomson Digital, Glen Vause

Contributors:
Robin Arnold, MSc, Ken Ashwell, BMedSc, MB, BS, PhD, Deborah Bryce, BSc, MScQual, MChiro,
GrCertHEd, John Gallo, MB, BS(Hons), FRACP, FRCPA, Rakesh Kumar, MB, BS, PhD, Peter Lavelle,
MB, BS, Karen McGhee, BSc, Michael Roberts, MB, BS, LLB(Hons), Emeritus Professor Frederick
Rost, BSc(Med), MB, BS, PhD, DCP(London), DipRMS, Elizabeth Tancred, BSc, PhD,Dzung Vu, MD,
MB, BS, DipAnat, GradCertHEd, Phil Waite, BSc(Hons), MBChB, CertHEd, PhD

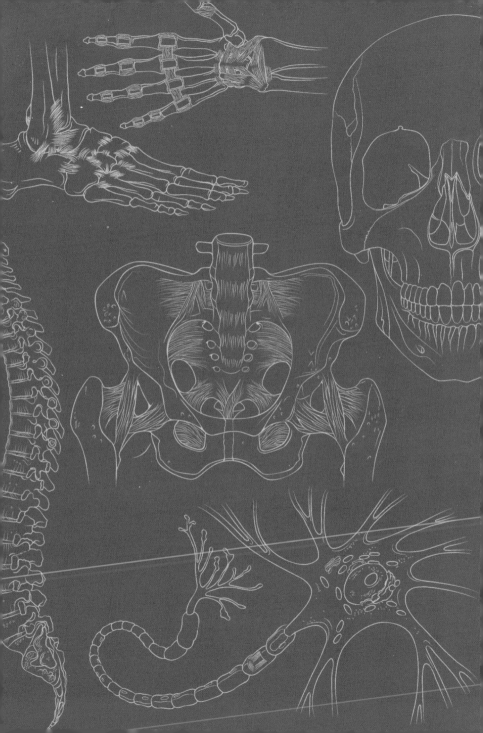

Contents

Joints

Introduction

There are two important principles embodied in this book. The first is that anatomy is a three-dimensional, fundamentally visual subject, which is best learned by the student using their hand and eye to follow the position, contours, and courses of bones, muscles, vessels, and nerves. Anatomy cannot be learned simply as textual information—for proper understanding of the structure of the human body, students must be able to hold the positions, relationships, and trajectories of anatomical structures in their "mind's eye."

The second is that learning in any field, but especially in anatomy, is most effective when it is an active process. Retention of knowledge is more complete when the student is actively involved in testing themselves against the body of knowledge they wish to retain. Passive immersion in a body of information by reading text will rarely lead to any significant retention of knowledge.

By combining these two important educational principles, this book provides an effective, convenient tool for students to master the important elements of human structure. Students are encouraged to use the book in conjunction with their recommended text to absorb and reinforce critically important concepts in the topography of the human body.

Ken Ashwell, BMedSc, MBBS, PhD
Professor of Anatomy,
Department of Anatomy,
School of Medical Sciences,
The University of New South Wales
Sydney, Australia

How to Use this Book

This book is designed to assist students and professionals to identify body parts and structures, and the numbered leader lines aid the process by clearly pointing out each body part. The function of coloring allows you to familiarize yourself with individual parts of the body and check your knowledge.

Coloring is best done using either pencils or pens in a variety of dark and light colors. Where possible, you should use the same color for like structures, so that all completed illustrations can be utilized later as visual references. According to anatomical convention, the color green is usually reserved for lymphatic structures, yellow for nerves, red for arteries, and blue for veins.

The numbered leader lines that point to separate parts of the illustration enable you to consolidate and then check your knowledge using the keys and descriptions on the facing page.

Body Regions

Key:

1 Head
2 Cranium (cranial)
3 Face (facial)
4 Mouth (oral)
5 Chin (mental)
6 Axilla (axillary)
7 Brachium (brachial)
8 Cubital fossa
9 Forearm (antebrachial)
10 Wrist (carpal)
11 Pollex (thumb)
12 Palm (palmar)
13 Digits (digital or phalangeal)
14 Inguen (inguinal)
15 Pubis (pubic)
16 Femur (femoral)
17 Patella (patellar)
18 Crus (crural)
19 Tarsus (tarsal)
20 Digits (digital or phalangeal)
21 Hallux (big toe)
22 Pes (pedal)
23 Hand (manual)
24 Pelvis (pelvic)
25 Umbilicus (umbilical)
26 Epigastrium (epigastric)
27 Thorax (thoracic)
28 Trunk
29 Neck (cervical)
30 Cheek (buccal)
31 Nose (nasal)
32 Orbit (orbital)
33 Forehead (frontal)
34 Ear (auricular)

Description:

Anatomists divide the surface of the body into different areas. The head contains the cranium and face. The trunk contains the thorax, abdomen, and pelvis. At the base of the pelvis are the inguinal and pubic regions. The upper limb is divided into axillary, brachial, antebrachial, and manual regions. The lower limb is divided into inguinal, femoral, crural, and pedal regions.

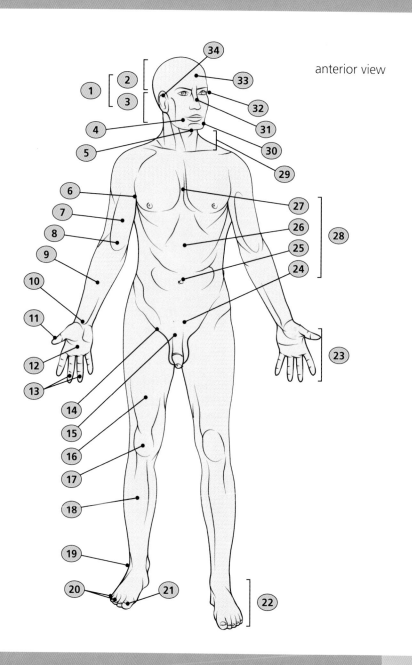

anterior view

Body Regions

Key:

1 Shoulder (acromial)
2 Back (dorsal)
3 Olecranon (olecranal)
4 Lower back (lumbar)
5 Gluteus (gluteal)
6 Popliteus (popliteal)
7 Sura (sural)
8 Calcaneus (calcaneal)
9 Sole (plantar)
10 Lower limb
11 Upper limb
12 Neck (cervical)
13 Head (cephalic)

Description:
The back and the gluteal regions are located posteriorly. Each upper limb consists of an arm, forearm, and hand. Each lower limb consists of a thigh, leg, and foot. Fossae—cavities or depressions in bone or body regions—are present anteriorly at the elbow (cubital fossa), and posteriorly at the knee (popliteal fossa).

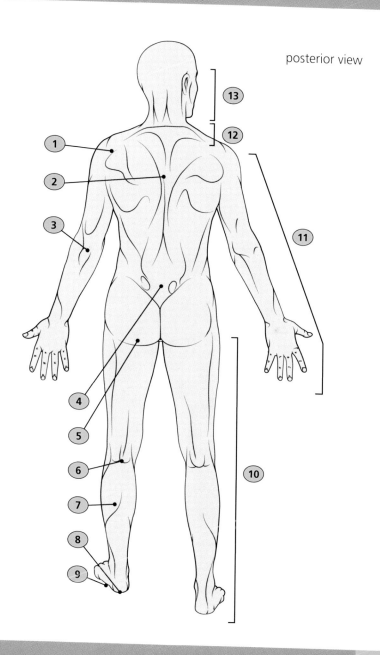

posterior view

Body Cavities

Key:

1 Torso or trunk

2 Thoracic cavity

3 Pericardial cavity

4 Abdominopelvic cavity

5 Diaphragm

6 Abdominal cavity

7 Pelvic cavity

8 Spinal canal

9 Cranial cavity

10 Dorsal cavity

Description:

The body cavities are spaces containing the internal organs (viscera). The main cavities are the thoracic and abdominopelvic cavities in the torso, and the cranial cavity in the head.

The thoracic (or chest) cavity contains the heart, lungs, trachea, and esophagus. The abdominopelvic cavity is divided into the abdominal cavity and pelvic cavity. The abdominal cavity contains most of the gastrointestinal tract, kidneys, and adrenal glands. Below the abdominal cavity, the pelvic cavity contains the urogenital system and the rectum. The cranial cavity contains the brain and extends caudally as the spinal canal.

sagittal view

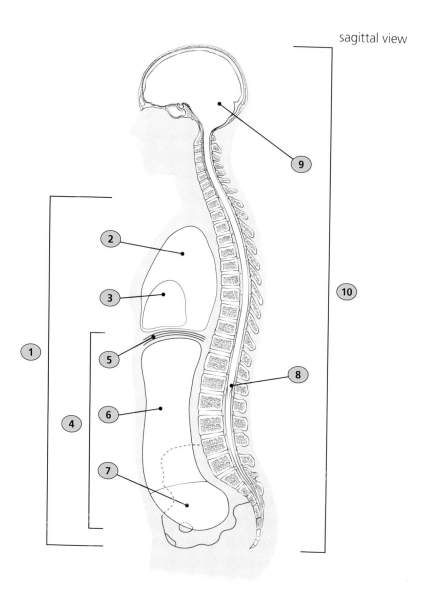

Anatomical Planes

Key:

1 Frontal (coronal) plane
2 Transverse (axial or horizontal) plane
3 Sagittal (midsagittal) plane
4 Parasagittal plane

Description:

Specific terms describe the orientation and relationships of the body and its parts. Sections of the body are described in terms of anatomical planes (flat surfaces). These are imaginary lines—vertical or horizontal—drawn through a body in the anatomical position (that is, with the body standing erect, feet together with toes pointed forward, and arms at the sides with palms facing forward). A frontal (coronal) plane divides the body into dorsal (posterior, or back) and ventral (anterior, or front) pieces. A transverse (axial or horizontal) plane cuts the body across from side to side, separating superior areas above from inferior areas below. A sagittal plane separates one side of the body from the other side (left from right). The midsagittal (median) plane is the sagittal plane exactly in the middle of the body.

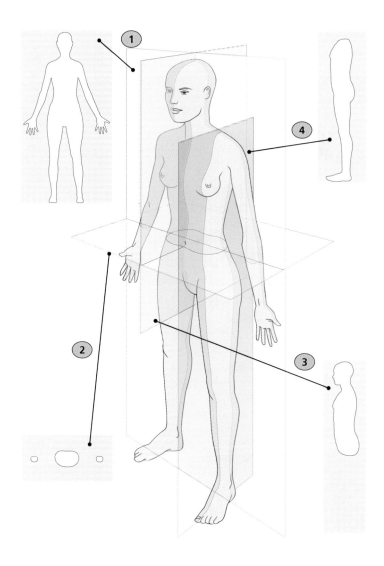

Anatomical View Orientation

Key:

1	Anterior	7	Palmar surface of hand
2	Proximal	8	Dorsal surface of hand
3	Distal	9	Lateral
4	Dorsal surface of foot	10	Posterior
5	Plantar surface of foot	11	Medial
6	Inferior	12	Superior

Description:

The relationships of one body part to another are identified by terms such as medial (toward the midline of the body) or lateral (away from the midline of the body); inferior (below, or lower) or superior (above, or upper); cranial (toward the head) or caudal (toward the tail); anterior (ventral, or toward the front) or posterior (dorsal, or toward the back); proximal (closer to a reference point) or distal (farther from that reference point).

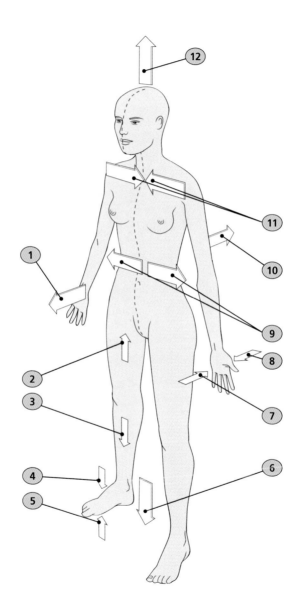

Cells and Tissues

The human body is made up of trillions of cells grouped into thousands of types. Despite this diversity, every cell has the same basic structure: a nucleus containing genetic material, a surrounding cytoplasm with organelles performing key functions, and an enclosing cell membrane to hold the structure together and regulate movement of nutrients and waste into and out of the cell. Cell types include body surface layer and glandular cells (epithelium of skin, gut lining, respiratory tract); contractile cells (muscle cells); information-processing cells (nerve cells); and connective tissue cells that make a surrounding matrix (bone, cartilage, fibrous tissue, fat, blood).

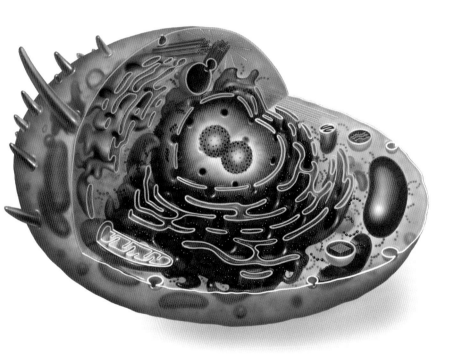

Cells and Tissues

Cell Structure

Key:

1 Nucleus
2 Golgi apparatus
3 Cilium
4 Microvilli
5 Location of chromatin
6 Mitochondrion
7 Cell membrane
8 Ribosome on endoplasmic
   reticulum

9 Peroxisome
10 Nucleolus
11 Cytoplasm
12 Nuclear pores
13 Lysosome
14 Centriole

Description:
Cells are the basic units of the body. Every adult body contains more than 5 trillion cells. Cells are surrounded by a cell membrane. Within the cell membrane lies the cytoplasm, a fluid containing many important structural units called organelles. These include rough endoplasmic reticulum, mitochondria, Golgi apparatus, and centrioles. The nucleus is separated from the cytoplasm by a nuclear membrane. Cells are specialized to perform particular functions.

microstructure

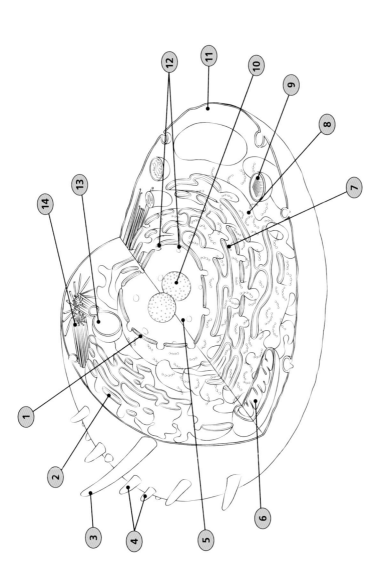

Neuron

Key:

1 Terminal bouton
2 Axon terminal
3 Axon
4 Myelin sheath
5 Dendrite
6 Mitochondrion
7 Nucleolus
8 Nucleus
9 Golgi apparatus
10 Cell body

Description:

Neurons are specialized cells that conduct nerve impulses. Each has three main parts—the cell body, branching processes (dendrites) that carry impulses to the cell body, and one elongated projection (axon) that conveys impulses away from the cell body. Neurons usually have a single axon, and a variable number of dendrites, depending on the cell's function.

microstructure

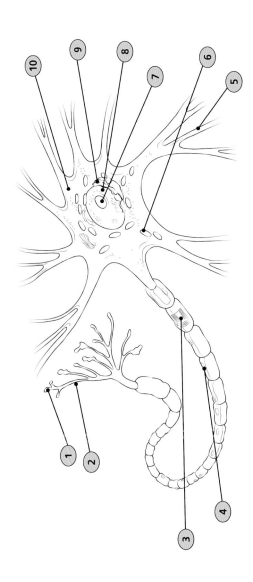

Loose Connective Tissue

Key:

1 Nerve
2 Adipose cell
3 Lymphocyte
4 Red blood cell
5 Capillary
6 Neutrophil
7 Mast cell
8 Monocyte
9 Areolar loose connective tissue

Description:
Tissue refers to a group or layer of cells, plus the material packed between them, all of which function together for the same specialized purpose. There are four major types of tissues in the body—connective, epithelial, neural, and muscular. Connective tissue is tissue made up of cells and protein fibers arranged in a framework that provides support for other body tissues and holds them together. Humans have five main types of connective tissue—loose connective tissue (including adipose tissue), dense connective tissue, cartilage, bone, and blood.

microstructure

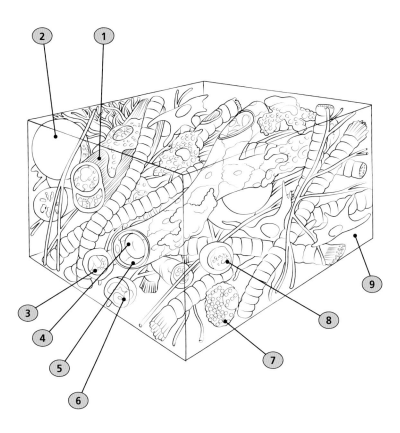

Muscle Tissue

Key:

1 Skeletal muscle tissue
2 Cardiac muscle tissue
3 Smooth muscle tissue

Description:

Muscle tissue is composed of cells that are purpose-built for contraction. There are three main forms—skeletal, cardiac, and smooth.

The muscle fibers, or myofibers, of skeletal muscle are long and cylindrical, arranged parallel to each other, and have a striped appearance under the microscope. Skeletal muscles allow the body to move. They are voluntary muscles, controlled by the brain and spinal cord.

Cardiac muscle cells are similar to skeletal muscle cells, as they also have a striped appearance. They, however, are branched. Cardiac muscle is the heart muscle, which contracts and relaxes rhythmically in an involuntary manner.

Smooth muscle tissue has no striations. Smooth muscle is controlled by the autonomic nervous system and is found in the skin, the blood vessels, and the reproductive and digestive systems.

microstructure

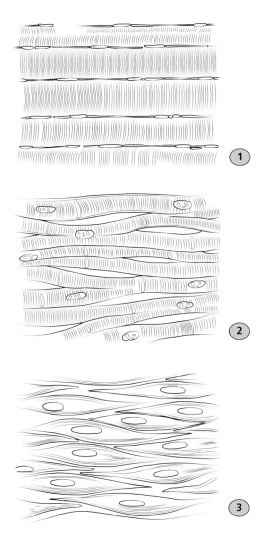

Skin

Key:

1 Epidermis
2 Dermis
3 Subcutaneous fat (hypodermis)
4 Sweat gland
5 Ruffini ending
6 Free nerve ending
7 Nerve ending
8 Krause bulb
9 Pacinian corpuscle

10 Dermal papilla
11 Deep fascia
12 Hair follicle
13 Sebaceous gland
14 Stratum spinosum
15 Stratum granulosum
16 Stratum corneum
17 Hair
18 Meissner corpuscles

Description:

Skin is composed of two layers. The outer layer, the epidermis or epithelium, is several cells thick. The deepest layers of the epidermis, the basal and spinous layers (stratum granulosum and stratum spinosum, respectively), are made up of living cells. These two layers produce keratinocytes, which contain the protein keratin. The outer layer of the epidermis, the horny layer (or stratum corneum), is made up of dead keratinocytes.

The dermis is the skin's inner layer and contains networks of blood vessels and nerves. Among the layers of the epidermis and the dermis are the hair follicles, the sweat glands, and the sebaceous glands. The skin is a protective organ that covers the body, merging with mucous membranes at the openings of the body, such as the mouth and the anus. Specialized nerve receptors in the skin allow the body to sense pain, heat and cold, touch, and pressure. Skin plays a role in temperature regulation, protection from ultraviolet light, and the manufacture of vitamin D.

microstructure

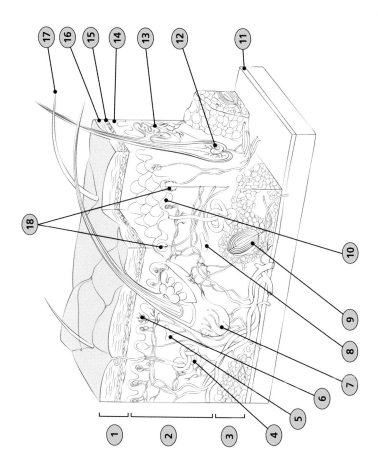

Cells and Tissues

Scalp and Hair

Scalp Key:

1 Hair
2 Hair follicle
3 Loose areolar tissue
4 Skull bone
5 Pericranium
6 Aponeurosis
7 Skin

Hair Key:

8 Epidermis
9 Precuticular epithelium
10 Internal root sheath
11 External root sheath
12 Nerve
13 Follicle sheath
14 Dermal hair papilla
15 Melanocyte
16 Hair bulb
17 Internal root sheath
18 External root sheath
19 Follicle sheath
20 Erector pili muscle (arrector pili)
21 Sebaceous gland
22 Medulla
23 Cortex
24 Cuticle
25 Hair shaft

Scalp Description:

The scalp is the skin and connective tissue covering the skull. The skin is attached to the skull by the loose areolar tissue and the pericranium.

The hair that grows from it protects against heat loss, minor abrasions, and ultraviolet light. The adult human scalp contains around 100,000 hair follicles.

Hair Description:

Hair is made of keratin and has a fine threadlike structure, consisting of a root, embedded in the skin; and a shaft, projecting from the skin surface. The root ends in a soft whitish enlargement, the hair bulb, which is lodged in an elongated pit in the skin called the follicle. Short fine hair covers most of the body, with some areas more densely covered.

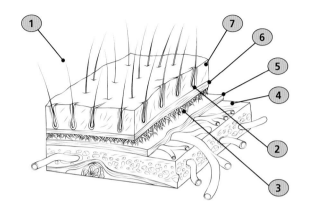

Scalp

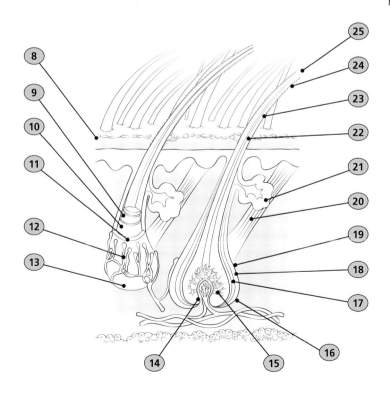

Hair

Skeletal System

The skeleton not only provides a protective framework for the body and sites for attachment of muscles, but is an important storage site for calcium and phosphate, and houses the blood-forming (hematopoietic) tissues of the body (red bone marrow). The remarkable rigidity and strength of bone come from its composite nature, blending mineral components (i.e., crystals of calcium hydroxyapatite) and organic components (e.g., collagen fibers). Bones come in a variety of sizes and shapes, from the tiny stapes (stirrup) of the middle ear cavity, to the weight-bearing tubular long bones of the thigh and leg (femur, tibia, and fibula).

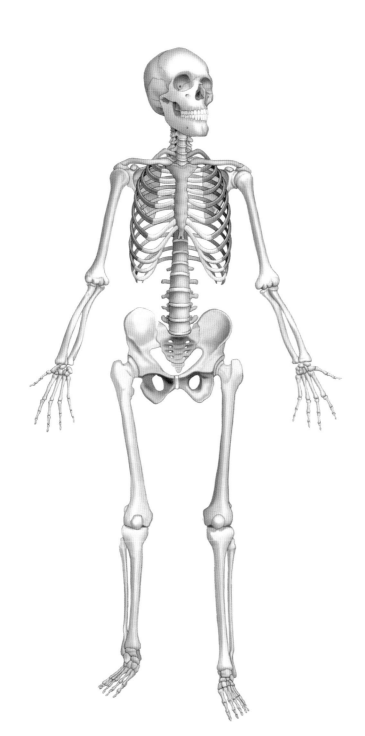

Skeletal System

Key:

1 Frontal bone	12 Twelfth rib (floating rib)
2 Parietal bone	13 Humerus
3 Temporal bone	14 Sternum
4 Maxilla	15 Clavicle
5 Cervical vertebra	16 Mandible
6 Costal cartilage	17 Lower teeth
7 True rib	18 Upper teeth
8 Thoracic vertebra	19 Anterior nasal (or piriform) aperture
9 False rib	20 Orbit
10 Lumbar vertebra	
11 Transverse process	

Description:

The skeleton is the framework of the body—supporting it and protecting the internal organs. The skeleton is usually described in two parts—the axial skeleton and the appendicular skeleton. The axial skeleton consists of the skull, vertebral column, and thoracic cage. The appendicular skeleton consists of the bones of the limbs and the shoulder and pelvic girdles.

Continued on page 38

anterior view

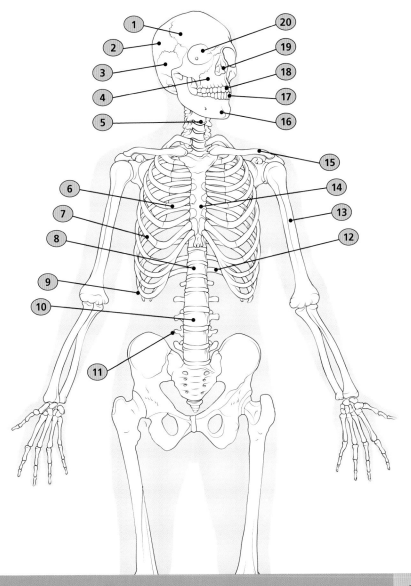

Skeletal System

Key:

1	Ilium	11	Tibia
2	Sacrum	12	Patella
3	Coccyx	13	Femur
4	Pubic symphysis	14	Body of pubis
5	Ischium	15	Phalanges
6	Tarsal bones	16	Metacarpal bone
7	Phalanges	17	Carpal bones
8	Metatarsal bone	18	Ulna
9	Talus	19	Radius
10	Fibula		

Continued from page 36

The skeletal system has intense weight-bearing responsibilities. Bone is rigid calcified tissue, which offers maximum strength without being too heavy. Wherever two bones come into contact with each other, there is a joint (or suture, for adjoining bones of the skull). The bones may be separated by cartilage, fluid, or fibrous tissue.

anterior view

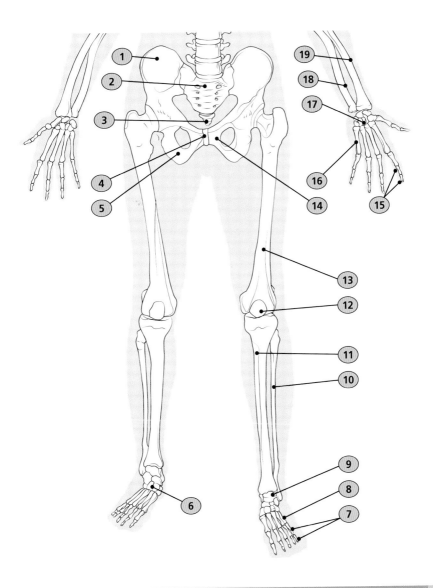

Skeletal System

Key:

1 Parietal bone
2 Occipital bone
3 Atlas (C1)
4 Axis (C2)
5 Cervical vertebra
6 Thoracic vertebra
7 Floating ribs (Pairs 11 & 12)
8 Lumbar vertebra
9 Ulna
10 Radius

11 False rib
12 True rib
13 Humerus
14 Scapula
15 Acromion
16 Spine of the scapula
17 Clavicle
18 Mandible
19 Zygomatic bone

Description:

The skeleton is the framework of the body and is usually described in two parts—the axial skeleton and the appendicular skeleton. The axial skeleton consists of the skull, the vertebral column, and the thoracic cage. The appendicular skeleton consists of the bones of the limbs and the shoulder and pelvic girdles.

Continued on page 42

posterior view

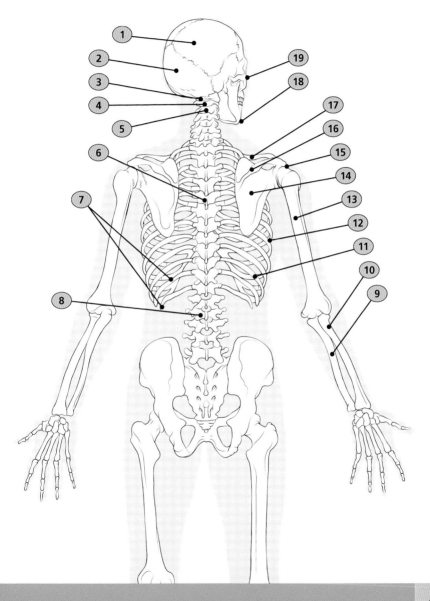

Skeletal System

Key:

1	Ilium	8	Calcaneus
2	Carpal bones	9	Talus
3	Metacarpal bones	10	Femoral condyle
4	Phalanges	11	Pubic symphysis
5	Femur	12	Ischial tuberosity
6	Tibia	13	Coccyx
7	Fibula	14	Sacrum

Continued from page 40

Wherever two bones come into contact, there is a joint (or suture, for adjoining bones of the skull). The bones may be separated by cartilage or fluid, such as is found in synovial joints. Some joints offer little movement, while the most mobile joints in the body are the synovial joints found in the appendicular skeleton.

posterior view

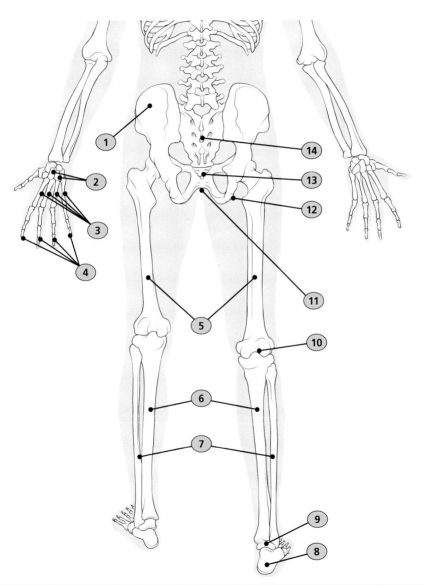

Skeletal System

Bone Structure

Key:

1 Muscle
2 Tendon
3 Epiphyseal plate
4 Marrow cavity
5 Bone marrow
6 Cortical bone
7 Periosteum
8 Inner circumferential lamella
9 Volkmann's canal

10 Interstitial lamellae
11 Outer circumferential lamellae
12 Concentric lamellae
13 Haversian canals
14 Trabecula of spongy bone
15 Endosteum
16 Spongy bone

Description:

Making up the skeleton, bone is a type of connective tissue, and, as such, is composed of cells in a matrix. The major components of the matrix include mineral salts (mainly calcium phosphate), which provide hardness, and collagen fibers, which give strength. Four types of cells are present —osteoprogenitor cells, osteoblasts, osteocytes, and osteoclasts. Osteoprogenitor cells develop into osteoblasts, which form bone tissue. Osteoblasts mature into osteocytes, which maintain bone tissue. Osteoclasts, which occur on bone surfaces, are involved in the reabsorption of the matrix, required for bone development, growth, and repair.

Bones act as a store of calcium and house the bone marrow in which blood cells are manufactured. A typical mature long bone has a central shaft—the diaphysis—and ends known as epiphyses. The diaphysis meets the epiphysis at the metaphysis. This is the location, in an immature bone, of the cartilage layer from which lengthwise growth occurs. Most of the bone is protected and nourished by the periosteum —a membrane served by nerves and blood vessels.

cross-sectional view of the proximal femur

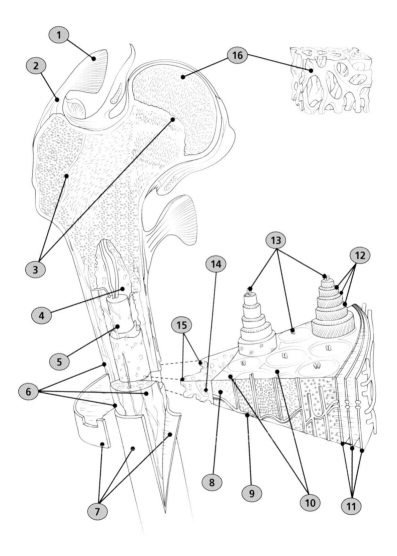

Bone Growth

Key:

1 Superficial layer of bone
2 Chondrocytes
3 Compact bone
4 Spongy bone
5 Secondary ossification centers (epiphyses)
6 Growth plate

Description:

Long bones begin as cartilage models in the embryo. Chondrocytes secrete cartilage matrix, leading to mature cartilage.

By birth, ossification (development of bone) has reached almost to the articular ends (epiphyses) of the cartilage models. New centers of bone growth also form in the articular ends of the developing long bones. A plate of cartilage (a growth plate) persists along the leading edge of ossification and is responsible for lengthening of the developing long bones. The growth plate moves steadily away from the center of the bone toward the ends until all the cartilage has ossified. Growth in bone length is then complete. By the age of about 20, ossification reaches and includes the growth plate, at which time growth stops.

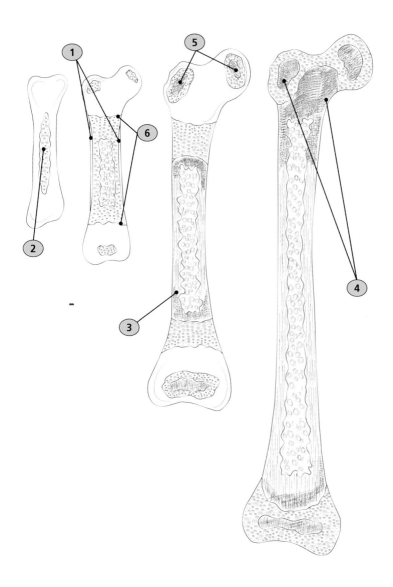

Bones of the Skull

Key:

1 Parietal bone
2 Lesser wing of sphenoid bone
3 Temporal bone
4 Greater wing of sphenoid bone
5 Nasal septum
6 Mental foramen
7 Mandible
8 Lower (mandibular) teeth
9 Upper (maxillary) teeth
10 Maxilla
11 Zygomatic bone
12 Nasal bone
13 Frontal bone

Description:

The skull forms the skeleton of the head and consists of the cranium and the mandible. The neurocranium surrounds and protects the brain and part of the brainstem. The facial cranium is the lower part of the skull that underlies the face. Fourteen bones make up the facial cranium, including the two nasal bones, forming the upper portion of the bridge of the nose; two lacrimal bones, which are located in each orbit (eye socket) next to the nose and close to the tear ducts; the maxillary bones (upper jaw); the mandible (lower jaw); the two palatine bones of the hard palate; the vomer, which, with a part of the ethmoid bone, makes up the nasal septum; and the two inferior turbinates of the nose.

The bones of the skull are linked together by joints known as sutures, which are found only in the skull—no active movement occurs at these joints. The adjacent bones have irregular interlocking edges bound together by fibrous connective tissue. The base of the skull articulates with the atlas (C1) of the vertebral column—this joint allows the head to flex and extend. The mandible articulates with the temporal bones on each side at the temporomandibular joint.

anterior view

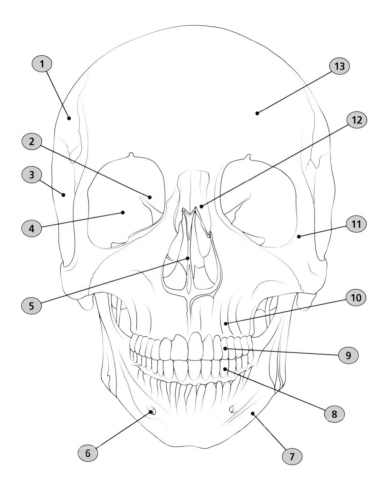

Bones of the Skull

Key:

1 Sagittal suture
2 Lambda
3 Temporal bone
4 Lambdoid suture
5 Mastoid process
6 Mandible
7 External occipital protuberance
8 Occipital bone
9 Parietal bone

Description:

The roof or vault of the neurocranium is formed by several major bones—the paired parietal and temporal bones, the frontal bone, and the occipital bone. The rear view of the skull is dominated by the occipital bone in the midline below, with the parietal bones above on each side. The cranial bones overlie the four correspondingly named lobes of the brain. The bones of the skull are connected by joints known as sutures. Though classed as joints, the connections between the skull bones are fixed and immobile.

posterior view

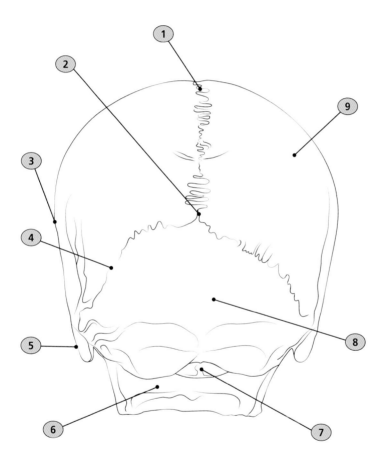

Bones of the Skull

Key:

1 Parietal bone
2 Lambdoid suture
3 Occipital bone
4 Mastoid process
5 Mandible
6 Mental foramen
7 Mental protuberance
8 Maxilla
9 External auditory meatus
10 Zygomatic process of temporal bone
11 Zygomatic bone
12 Nasal bone
13 Lacrimal bone
14 Ethmoid bone
15 Greater wing of sphenoid bone
16 Squamous part of temporal bone
17 Frontal bone
18 Coronal suture

Description:

The cranial bones—occipital, parietal, frontal, temporal, sphenoid, and ethmoid bones—provide a protective housing for the brain, while the remaining 14 bones of the skull give form to the facial features. In a lateral view, the division of the skull into the larger ovoid brain case (neurocranium) and the smaller triangular face (facial cranium) is evident. The orbits are pyramidal spaces (tapering posteriorly) on either side of the face. At the sides of the skull, the temporal bones contain a system of spaces, which form the middle and inner parts of the ears. Within the middle ear are the auditory ossicles—the malleus, incus, and stapes.

The cranial bones meet at sutures, which are fixed and immobile joints. The mandible articulates with the two temporal bones on each side at the temporomandibular joint. These joints are condyloid synovial joints, enabling the mandible to be elevated and depressed, protruded, retracted, and moved from side to side.

lateral view

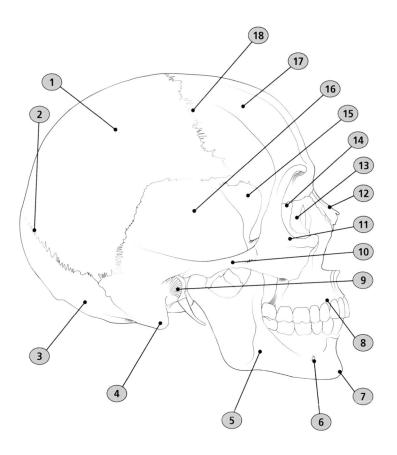

Bones of the Skull

Key:

1 Petrous part of temporal bone
2 Parietal bone
3 Lambdoid suture
4 Occipital bone
5 Mandibular foramen
6 Medial pterygoid plate
7 Mylohyoid line of mandible
8 Maxilla
9 Perpendicular plate of ethmoid bone
10 Nasal bone
11 Frontal sinus
12 Crista galli (ethmoid)
13 Frontal bone
14 Coronal suture

Description:

A sagittal view of the skull reveals the interrelationship of the bones of both the neurocranium and the facial cranium. The bones of the skull enclose several spaces. The largest cavity accommodates the brain; this is usually described as three contiguous regions—the anterior, middle, and posterior cranial fossae. The nasal cavities are flattened chambers, into which protrude curved plates called conchae or turbinates, which increase the surface area of the nasal cavities. The nasal cavities are connected to paranasal sinuses in the frontal, ethmoid, maxillary, and sphenoid bones. The maxillary sinuses, which lie to the sides of the nose, are the largest.

Each side of the mandible has a head that fits into a socket in the temporal bone of the skull, forming the temporomandibular joint. The four major bones of the neurocranium—the occipital, parietal, temporal, and frontal bones—join at sutures, which are bound together by fibrous connective tissue.

sagittal view

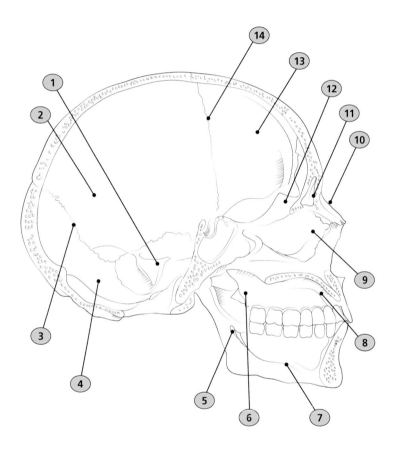

Bones of the Skull: Base of the Skull

Key:

1 Zygomatic bone
2 Greater wing of sphenoid bone
3 Vomer
4 Occipital condyle
5 Foramen magnum
6 Occipital bone
7 External occipital protuberance
8 Mastoid process
9 Styloid process
10 Mandibular fossa
11 Lateral pterygoid plate
12 Zygomatic arch
13 Medial pterygoid plate
14 Posterior nasal aperture
15 Horizontal plate of palatine bone
16 Palatine process (maxilla)

Description:

A number of bones, both neurocranial and facial cranial, come together to form the base of the skull. The base of the skull contains a number of foramina, through which the spinal cord, cranial nerves, and blood vessels enter or exit.

The base of the skull articulates with the atlas (C1), the first cervical vertebra of the vertebral column.

inferior view

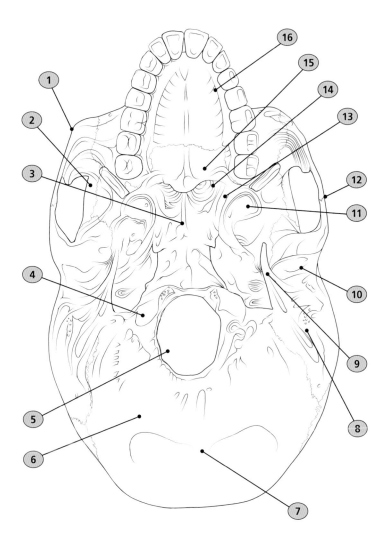

Fetal Skull Development: Prenatal

Key:

1	Frontal bone	13	Nasal bone
2	Nasal bone	14	Maxilla
3	Maxilla	15	Mandible
4	Zygomatic bone	16	Styloid process
5	Mandible	17	Mastoid part of temporal bone
6	Styloid process		
7	Tympanic ring	18	Tympanic ring
8	Squamous part of temporal bone	19	Zygomatic process
		20	Squamous part of temporal bone
9	Squamous part of occipital bone		
		21	Temporal bone
10	Parietal eminence	22	Occipital bone
11	Parietal bone	23	Parietal bone
12	Frontal bone		

Description:

Development and growth occur in the uterus, from fertilization to formation of the embryo and the fetus to birth. During the embryonic stage, either cartilage or membrane derived from mesenchyme is laid down in the developing head, becoming a template for the skull. The base of the skull develops from cartilage, which gradually becomes ossified (bony) as bone spreads out from ossification centers in the cartilage. By 12 weeks of gestation, cartilage has been laid down and has become the base for the skull; and by 16 weeks of gestation, bone spreads out from the ossification centers in the other cartilages and membranous templates.

12 weeks—lateral view

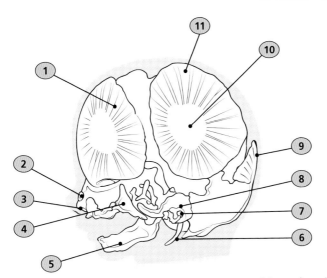

16 weeks—lateral view

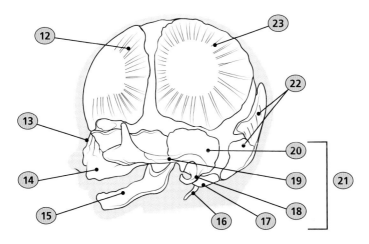

Fetal Skull Development: Full Term

Key:

1 Anterior fontanelle
2 Frontal bone
3 External acoustic meatus
4 Occipital bone
5 Parietal bone
6 Pterion
7 Anterior fontanelle
8 Metopic suture

9 Frontal bone
10 Coronal suture
11 Parietal bone
12 Lambdoid suture
13 Occipital bone
14 Posterior fontanelle
15 Sagittal suture

Description:

By full term, the skull is ossified, except for the fontanelles, which ossify after birth.

The fontanelle is a gap between the bones due to the normal delay in the joining together of several flat bones making up the skull. There are two fontanelles—the anterior located at the top of the skull, and the posterior, which is smaller and located at the back of the skull. The anterior fontanelle is commonly known as "the fontanelle." Normal closure of the gap occurs by about one year.

lateral view

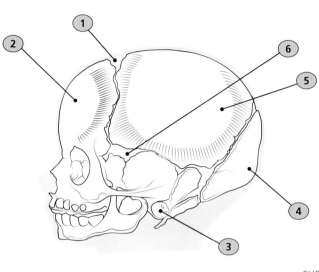

superior view

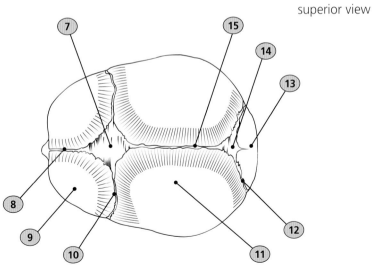

Orbital Cavity

Key:

1 Frontal bone
2 Temporal bone
3 Ethmoid bone
4 Cribriform plate of ethmoid bone
5 Eyeball
6 Frontal sinus

Description:

The frontal, ethmoid, lacrimal, zygomatic, nasal, palatine, sphenoid, and maxillary bones unite to form the orbit. The bones that form the outer wall and roof of the orbit are thick and strong, protecting the eye from injury, whereas the bones that form the inner walls are thin and fragile.

The bones that form the orbital cavity are united at sutures—immobile joints held firmly in place by fibrous connective tissue.

superior view

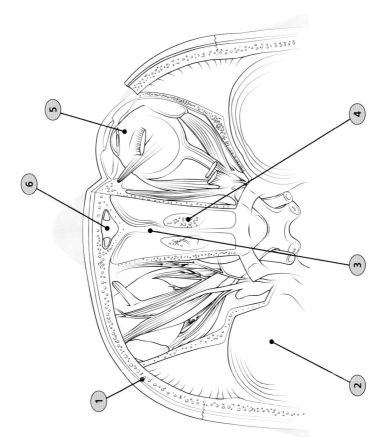

Skeletal System

Ear and Auditory Ossicles

Ear Key:
1 Temporal bone
2 Eustachian (auditory) tube
3 Cochlea
4 Stapes
5 Incus
6 Head of malleus
7 Tympanic membrane (eardrum)

Auditory Ossicles Key:
8 Head of malleus
9 Incus
10 Stapes
11 Posterior crus of stapes
12 Footplate of stapes
13 Anterior crus of stapes

Ear Description:
Located at the sides of the skull, the temporal bones contain the middle and inner ears. The middle ear contains a chain of three tiny bones that relay sound vibrations from the tympanic membrane (eardrum).

The auditory ossicles join to each other by synovial joints and work in unison, articulating in turn to transmit sound waves to the cochlea and acting as an amplifier by magnifying the movement of the eardrum. When the eardrum vibrates, the malleus vibrates the incus, which in turn vibrates the stapes. The base (or footplate) of the stapes covers the oval window, a membrane that passes vibrations into the spiral of the cochlea.

Auditory Ossicles Description:
The smallest bones in the body, the auditory ossicles of the middle ear have three members—the malleus, incus, and stapes (commonly known as the hammer, anvil, and stirrup, respectively). Vibrations generated at the eardrum are transmitted along this chain of bones, which connects across the tympanic cavity, to the oval window in the cochlea of the ear.

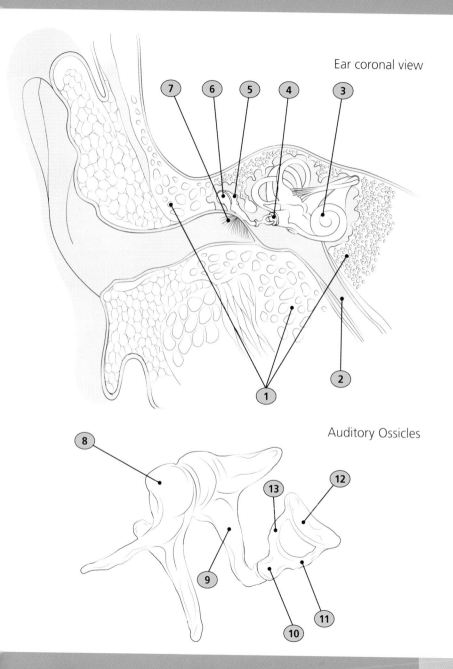

Ear coronal view

Auditory Ossicles

Vertebral Column

Lateral View Key:
1 Cervical vertebrae (C1–C7)
2 Thoracic vertebrae (T1–T12)
3 Lumbar vertebrae (L1–L5)
4 Sacrum
5 Coccyx
6 Intervertebral disks

Posterior View Key:
7 Cervical region (C1–C7)
8 Thoracic region (T1–T12)
9 Lumbar region (L1–L5)
10 Sacral region (S1–S5)
11 Coccygeal region
12 Transverse processes
13 Spinous processes
14 Axis (C2)
15 Atlas (C1)

Description:

The vertebral column is a chain of irregular bones called vertebrae. There are seven cervical vertebrae in the neck, twelve thoracic vertebrae in the chest, five lumbar vertebrae in the lower back, five fused bones that form the sacrum of the pelvis, and four fused bones that form the coccyx (vestigial tailbone). The vertebrae articulate with one another through intervertebral disks and zygapophyseal joints. Each vertebra can only move a few degrees at its intervertebral disk, but the sum of these individual movements gives mobility to the vertebral column. The twelve thoracic vertebrae all have ribs attached to their sides.

Each vertebra forms three separate joints with the vertebra above or below—a pair of facet joints (zygapophyseal joints) and a single anterior intervertebral joint. Movements of the vertebral column are flexion (to bend forward), lateral flexion (to bend sideways), extension (to bend backward), rotation (around its own axis), and circumduction (a combination of all these movements).

lateral view—left side

posterior view

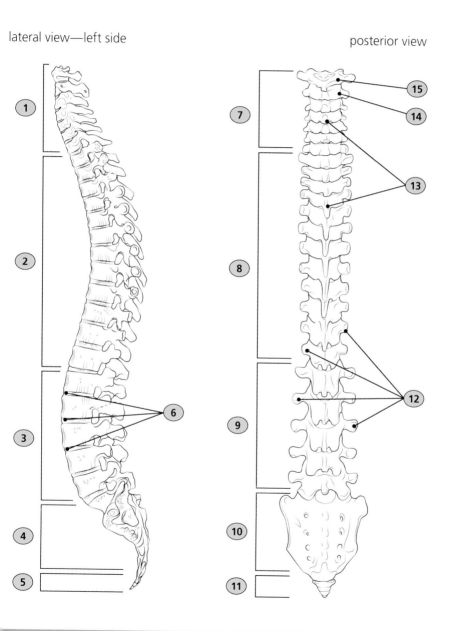

Cervical Vertebrae: Atlas (C1) and Axis (C2)

Cervical Vertebrae: Atlas (C1) Key:
1 Anterior tubercle
2 Anterior arch
3 Articular facet for dens
4 Vertebral foramen
5 Posterior arch
6 Posterior tubercle
7 Superior articular facet
8 Transverse foramen
9 Transverse process

Cervical Vertebrae: Axis (C2) Key:
10 Transverse process of axis
11 Transverse foramen
12 Inferior articular process
13 Spinous process
14 Vertebral foramen
15 Body of axis
16 Dens of axis
17 Superior articular facet
18 Facet for atlas

Cervical Vertebrae: Atlas (C1) Description:
The same basic elements are found in most vertebrae—a vertebral body, a vertebral arch comprising two pedicles and two laminae, and processes that project away from the arch. The bodies lie in front and are weight-bearing. They increase in size as they progress down the spine. The pedicles form the side walls of the vertebral foramen (spinal canal), and the two laminae form the back walls. The atlas and axis are specialized vertebrae. The first cervical vertebra, the atlas (C1), is a bony ring—unlike the other vertebrae, it does not have a body or spinous process.

Cervical Vertebrae: Axis (C2) Description:
The axis (C2) sits beneath the atlas, forming a pivot joint (the atlantoaxial joint) where the two vertebrae meet. The axis (C2) has an upward-projecting bony element known as the dens, which forms a joint in the midline with the atlas. This joint, together with a joint on either side, allows a pivoting movement to occur, as in shaking the head when saying no. About 45 degrees of rotation in the neck occurs at these joints alone.

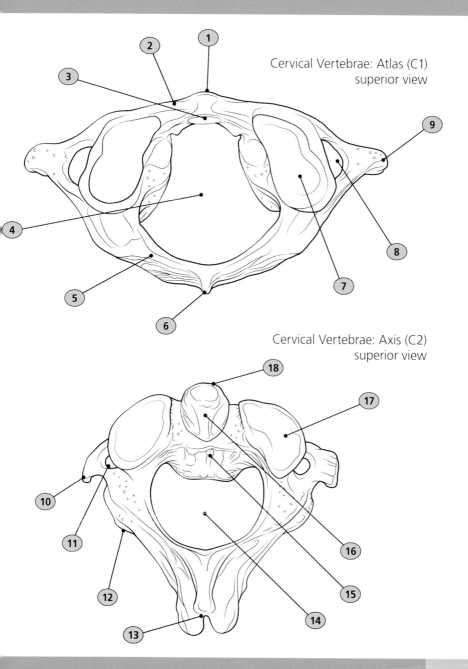

Cervical Vertebrae: Atlas (C1)
superior view

Cervical Vertebrae: Axis (C2)
superior view

Typical Cervical Vertebra

Key:

1 Body
2 Transverse foramen
3 Pedicle
4 Lamina
5 Vertebral foramen
6 Spinous process
7 Inferior articular process (facet)
8 Sulcus for ventral ramus of spinal nerve

9 Body
10 Transverse process
11 Superior articular process (facet)
12 Posterior tubercle of transverse process
13 Anterior tubercle of transverse process

Description:

There are seven cervical vertebrae (C1–C7). C1 and C2 are known as the atlas and axis, respectively, and are uniquely shaped. The remaining cervical vertebrae are similar in structure to most other vertebrae, and have a body, a vertebral arch comprising two pedicles and two laminae, and transverse processes that project away from the arch.

Each vertebra forms three separate joints with the vertebra above or below—a pair of facet joints and a single anterior intervertebral joint. The articular processes project up and down from the left and right sides of the vertebral arch and form facet joints with the articular processes of adjacent vertebrae. The orientation of these joint surfaces affects the direction of movement between vertebrae.

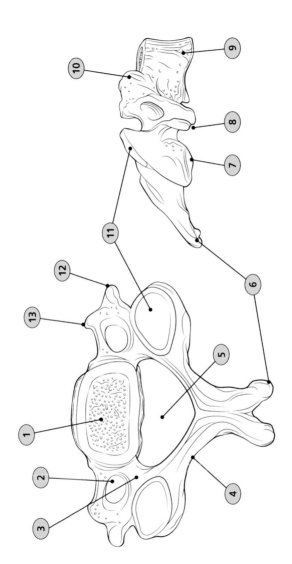

lateral view

superior view

Thoracic Vertebra

Key:
1 Pedicle, superior notch
2 Lamina
3 Spinous process
4 Inferior articular process (facet)
5 Inferior costal demifacet
6 Body
7 Superior costal demifacet
8 Superior articular process (facet)
9 Transverse costal facet

Description:
As with the majority of the vertebrae, each of the thoracic vertebrae features a similar structure, comprising a body, a vertebral arch, a spinous process, a pair of transverse processes, and two pairs of articular processes. Lying between the cervical and lumbar regions, the thoracic region of the vertebral column is formed by 12 vertebrae (T1–T12), all of which have ribs attached to their sides. The presence of the ribs and the orientation of the zygapophyseal (facet) joints means that the thoracic vertebrae have less range of movement than the neighboring groups of vertebrae.

The articular processes project up and down from the left and right sides of the vertebral arch and form joints, known as facet joints, with the articular processes of adjacent vertebrae. The facet joints are synovial joints held together by a joint capsule. The adjacent cartilage-covered surfaces are able to glide on each other during movements of the vertebral column. Synovial joints also occur between the 12 thoracic vertebrae and their connected ribs.

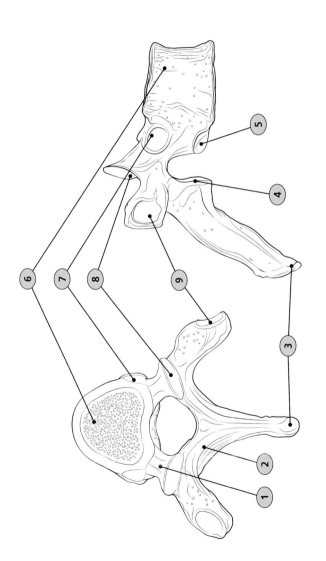

lateral view

superior view

Lumbar Vertebra

Key:

1 Superior articular process (facet)
2 Lamina
3 Spinous process
4 Inferior articular process (facet)
5 Pedicle
6 Body
7 Vertebral foramen
8 Pedicle
9 Mammillary process
10 Transverse process

Description:

The lumbar (lower back) region of the vertebral column has five vertebrae (L1–L5). The lumbar vertebrae are the largest of the vertebrae, to cope with their weight-bearing responsibility.

The articular processes of the lumbar vertebrae project up and down from the left and right sides of the vertebral arch and form joints with the articular processes of adjacent vertebrae. The orientation of these joint surfaces affects the direction of movement between vertebrae. Anterior intervertebral joints occur between the bodies of adjacent vertebrae.

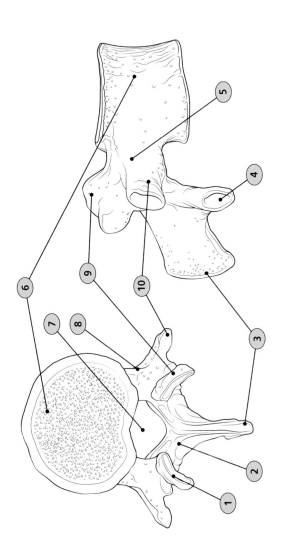

lateral view

superior view

Sacrum and Coccyx

Anterior View Key:
1 Sacral promontory
2 Anterior (ventral) sacral foramina
3 Coccyx
4 Sacrococcygeal joint

Posterior View Key:
5 Superior articular processes (facets)
6 Median sacral crest and spinous processes
7 Coccyx
8 Posterior (dorsal) sacral foramina

Anterior View Description:

The sacrum lies at the lower end of the spine beneath the lumbar vertebrae and forms part of the bony pelvis. A single curved bone in the adult, the sacrum actually develops from five separate vertebrae (S1–S5), which fuse to each other during early development to form a single bone. The spinal roots (cauda equina) of the spinal cord pass through the sacral canal, giving off sacral spinal nerves, which leave through the sacral foramina.

Posterior View Description:

The posterior view of the sacrum and coccyx shows the bony landmarks of the median sacral crest and the spinous tubercles. Dorsal sacral foramina perforate the surface of the sacrum. Both the sacrum and coccyx are formed from fused vertebrae, with the sacrum comprising five fused vertebrae, and the coccyx comprising four fused vertebrae. This fusion takes place during development and is usually complete by the time a person reaches their late twenties.

The sacrum articulates with the final lumbar vertebra (L5) above; at each side with the ilium of the pelvis to form the sacroiliac joints; and with the coccyx below to form the sacrococcygeal joint.

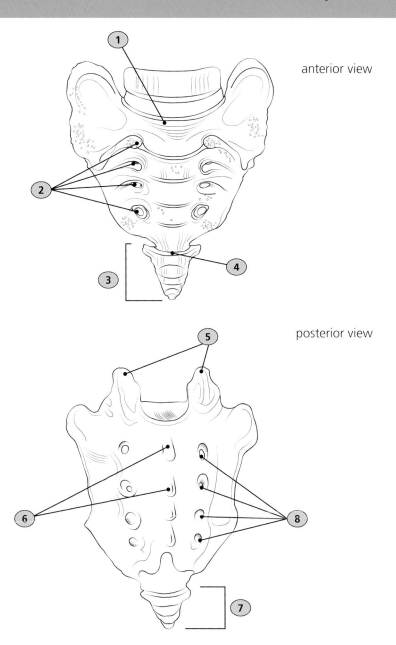

anterior view

posterior view

Rib Cage

Key:

1 Manubrium of sternum
2 Clavicle
3 Costal cartilage
4 Costochondral joint
5 Sternocostal joint
6 Xiphoid process

7 Body of sternum
8 False ribs (pairs 8–10)
9 True ribs (pairs 1–7)
10 Sternal angle
11 Sternoclavicular joint
12 Jugular notch

Description:

There are 12 pairs of ribs. Pairs 1–7 are known as "true ribs" because they connect directly through a costal cartilage to the sternum. From the thoracic vertebrae at the back, these ribs span around to the front, where they are joined to the sternum by costal cartilage. Pairs 8–10 are known as "false ribs," and they span around from the vertebrae at the back. However, the "false ribs" do not connect directly through a costal cartilage to the sternum. Instead, they are joined by costal cartilages to the seventh costal cartilage. Pairs 11–12 are known as "floating ribs," because they do not attach to the sternum at all, either directly or indirectly. These two pairs of ribs do not extend fully around to the front of the chest. Situated centrally in the thorax, the sternum (or breastbone) has three parts—the manubrium at the top, the body of the sternum in the middle, and the xiphoid process at the base. The "true ribs" are joined directly to the manubrium and the body of the sternum.

The manubrium articulates with the clavicles at the sternoclavicular joints. Joints are also found at the point where the costal cartilage of each rib joins the sternum (sternocostal joints), and where the costal cartilage joins the rib (costochondral joints).

anterior view

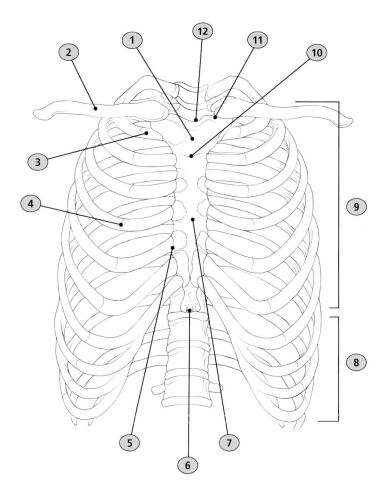

Skeletal System

Rib Cage

Key:
1 First thoracic vertebra (T1)
2 True ribs (pairs 1–7)
3 Lowest thoracic vertebra (T12)
4 Floating ribs (pairs 11–12)
5 False ribs (pairs 8–10)

Description:
The thoracic cage is made up of the 12 thoracic vertebrae (T1–T12), the ribs, and the sternum. The top seven true ribs (pairs 1–7) extend from the vertebrae at the back to the sternum at the front. The next three ribs (pairs 8–10) do not extend all the way around to the sternum, but instead connect by costal cartilage to the costal cartilage of the last true rib. The final two ribs (pairs 11–12), known as floating ribs, do not reach the front.

At the back, each rib articulates with its corresponding thoracic vertebra. At the front, the true ribs (pairs 1–7) articulate with the sternum.

posterior view

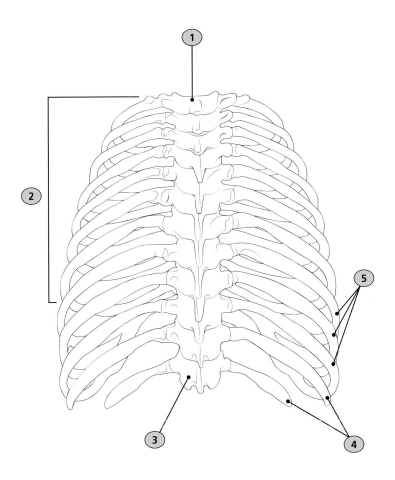

Skeletal System

Bones of the Upper Limb

Key:

1 Clavicle
2 Humerus
3 Radius
4 Ulna
5 Carpal bones
6 Metacarpal bones
7 Phalanges
8 Scapula (infraspinous fossa)
9 Spine of scapula
10 Acromion (of scapula)

Description:

The arm of the upper limb extends from the shoulder, where it is attached to the trunk, to the elbow, where it articulates with the ulna. The forearm extends from the elbow to the wrist, and contains the ulna and radius. The whole limb is designed for mobility, and gives the hand such a range of movement that it can reach most regions of the body and manipulate external objects.

The humerus attaches to the scapula (shoulder blade) at the shoulder joint. This is a ball-and-socket joint, in which the head of the humerus engages with a shallow socket on the shoulder blade. The shape of the joint gives mobility to the upper limb. The humerus articulates with the two forearm bones—the ulna and radius—at the elbow. The joint between the humerus and ulna is a synovial hinge joint and allows the arm to flex (bend) and extend. The ulna and radius articulate with the carpal bones at the wrist, to provide a range of movements.

anterior view—left limb

posterior view—right limb

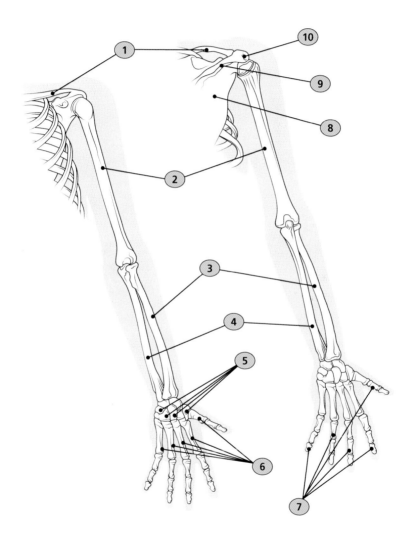

Clavicles

Key:

1 Clavicles
2 Manubrium (of sternum)
3 Sternoclavicular joint
4 Acromion (of scapula)
5 Acromioclavicular joint

Description:

The clavicles are a pair of short horizontal bones above the rib cage. The clavicles are attached to the sternum and the acromion of each scapula. The function of the clavicle is to stabilize the shoulder joint.

The acromioclavicular joint is formed where the acromion of the scapula meets the distal end of the clavicle. This joint allows a small amount of gliding movement to occur between the two bones in conjunction with movements of the arm. The acromioclavicular joint is supported by a capsule and several ligaments, the most important of which is the coracoclavicular ligament. These ligaments, which pass down from the undersurface of the clavicle to the coracoid process, also help to support the weight of the arm.

The point where the clavicle meets the manubrium of the sternum is the sternoclavicular joint. Held firm by ligaments, this joint plays a role in movements of the shoulder.

anterior view

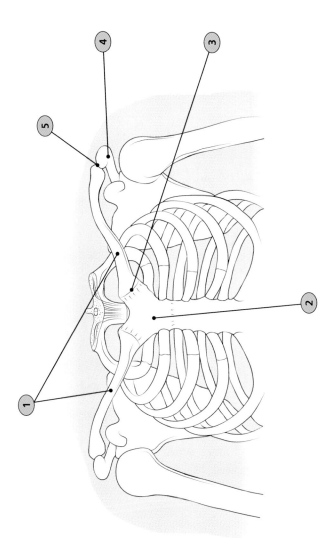

Shoulder Joint

Key:

1 Clavicle
2 Spine of scapula
3 Medial border (of scapula)
4 Lateral border (of scapula)
5 Glenoid fossa
6 Humerus (shaft)
7 Head of humerus
8 Acromion (of scapula)
9 Acromioclavicular joint
10 Coracoid process (of scapula)

Description:
The shoulder involves three bones—the clavicle, scapula, and humerus. The clavicle and scapula form the pectoral girdle, responsible for the attachment of the upper limb to the trunk. The clavicle acts as a strut to hold the upper limb away from the center of the body. The scapula is a flat triangular-shaped bone that covers part of the upper back. Together, the scapula and humerus form the highly mobile shoulder joint. A multiaxial ball-and-socket joint, the shoulder joint is capable of movement in almost any direction.

Joints are formed where the humerus and scapula meet (shoulder joint, or glenohumeral joint), and where the acromion and clavicle meet (acromioclavicular joint).

posterior view

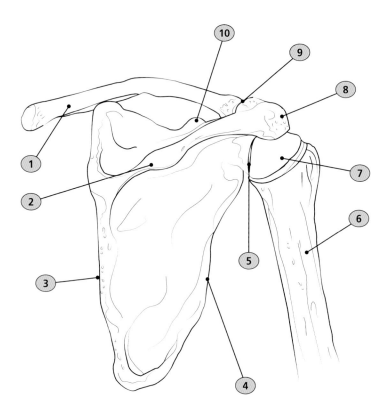

Humerus

Key:

1. Greater tubercle
2. Head of humerus
3. Anatomical neck
4. Lesser tubercle
5. Intertubercular sulcus
6. Surgical neck
7. Deltoid tuberosity
8. Radial groove
9. Lateral supracondylar ridge
10. Medial supracondylar ridge
11. Olecranon fossa
12. Coronoid fossa
13. Medial epicondyle
14. Trochlea
15. Capitulum
16. Lateral epicondyle
17. Radial fossa

Description:

The humerus consists of a cylindrical shaft, with a rounded head at its proximal end, and paired condyles at its distal end. Other landmarks of the humerus include the deltoid tuberosity, which is the point of attachment for the deltoid muscle; the medial and lateral epicondyles, which are also points of attachment for muscles; and the trochlea, which articulates with the ulna to produce elbow movement.

The rounded head of the humerus articulates with the scapula at the glenoid fossa to form the shoulder joint. At its distal end, the capitulum and trochlea articulate with the radius and ulna, respectively, to form the elbow joint.

anterior view

posterior view

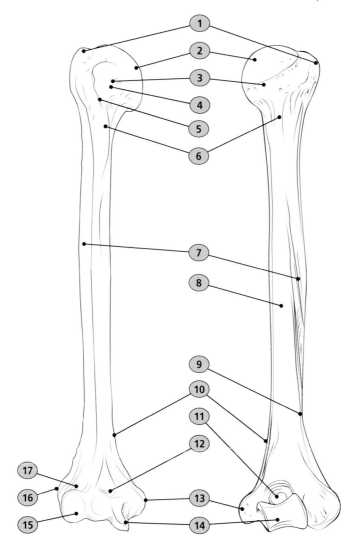

Skeletal System

Radius and Ulna

Key:

1 Olecranon
2 Trochlear notch
3 Proximal radioulnar joint
4 Coronoid process
5 Head of radius
6 Neck of radius
7 Ulnar tuberosity

8 Radial tuberosity
9 Ulna
10 Radius
11 Distal radioulnar joint
12 Head of ulna
13 Styloid process of ulna
14 Styloid process of radius

Description:
The radius is one of the two bones of the forearm. It is located on the thumb side, lying parallel to and rotating around the ulna. Near the uppermost end of the radius is a raised and roughened area called the radial tuberosity. At its larger distal end, the radius forms part of the wrist. The ulna lies on the medial side of the forearm, extending from the elbow to the wrist. The ulna is a long bone of irregular cross section, thickest at the proximal end and tapering toward the distal end. It projects above and behind the elbow.

anterior view

posterior view

Bones of the Wrist and Hand

Key:

1	Distal phalanges	8	Ulna
2	Middle phalanges	9	Lunate
3	Proximal phalanges	10	Triquetral
4	Trapezoid	11	Capitate
5	Trapezium	12	Hamate
6	Scaphoid	13	Metacarpal bones
7	Radius		

Description:

The wrist (carpus) is made up of eight carpal bones, which join the forearm to the hand. The bones of the hand consist of five metacarpal bones. Each of the four fingers (digits 2–5) contains three bones (the proximal, middle, and distal phalanges), while the thumb (digit 1) has two bones (the proximal and distal phalanges). The complex wrist joint allows a wide range of movement.

The joints formed between the radius and articular disk of the radioulnar joint of the forearm and the carpal bones of the wrist are ellipsoidal joints, while the carpal bones articulate with one another as gliding joints. The metacarpal bones then meet with the proximal phalanges of the fingers at the metacarpophalangeal (MCP) joints. Joints also exist between each of the adjoining phalanges.

dorsal view—right limb

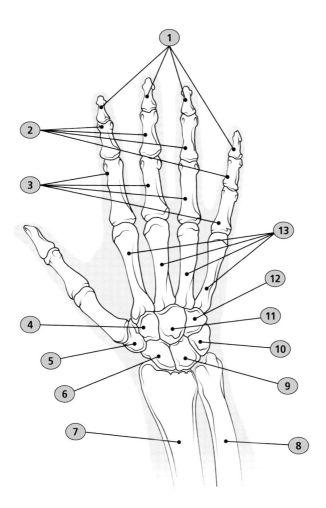

Bones of the Wrist and Hand

Key:

1	Distal phalanges	9	Scaphoid
2	Proximal phalanges	10	Capitate
3	Hamate	11	Trapezium
4	Triquetral	12	Trapezoid
5	Pisiform	13	Metacarpal bones
6	Lunate	14	Distal phalanx of thumb
7	Ulna	15	Middle phalanges
8	Radius		

Description:

The hand consists of the palm, the dorsum, and the thumb and fingers. Between the carpal bones of the wrist and the bones of the fingers (phalanges) are five metacarpal bones. The metacarpal bones join the phalanges at the metacarpophalangeal (MCP) joints, which are condylar in type, allowing flexion, extension, adduction, and abduction.

The phalanges in each finger meet at interphalangeal joints. Gliding joints occur between adjoining carpal bones of the wrist, and more hinge joints are formed where the carpal bones meet with the second to fifth metacarpal bones of the hand. At the thumb, a particularly mobile saddle joint is formed between the scaphoid bone of the wrist and the first metacarpal, allowing a wide range of movements.

palmar view—right limb

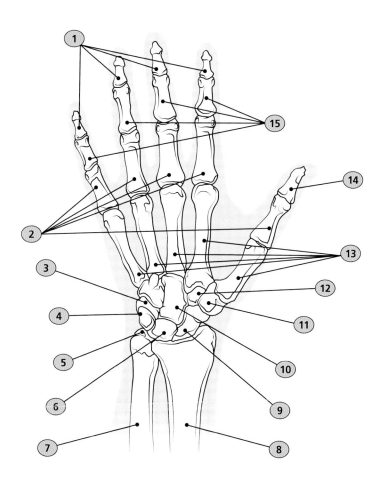

Finger

Key:

1 Proximal interphalangeal joint
2 Middle phalanx
3 Capsule
4 Articular cartilage
5 Fingernail
6 Distal phalanges

7 Distal interphalangeal joint
8 Proximal phalanges
9 Metacarpophalangeal joint
10 Metacarpal bones
11 Carpometacarpal joint
12 Carpal bones

Description:

Each finger has three bones (phalanges), separated by joints, except the thumb, which has only two phalanges. Fingernails, made mainly of the tough protein keratin, are designed to protect the sensitive tip of each finger. Interphalangeal joints occur between each of the phalanges of the finger. The interphalangeal joints are hinge joints, allowing movement in one plane only.

medial view

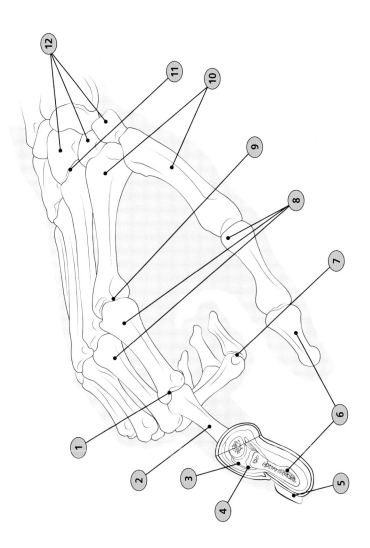

Bones of the Pelvis: Male

Key:

1 Iliac crest
2 Anterior superior iliac spine
3 Anterior inferior iliac spine
4 Superior pubic ramus
5 Pectineal line
6 Ischium
7 Pubic tubercle
8 Pubic symphysis
9 Inferior pubic ramus
10 Coccyx
11 Obturator foramen
12 Iliopectineal eminence
13 Sacrum
14 Alar part of sacrum
15 Sacral promontory
16 Ilium
17 Sacroiliac joint

Description:

The bony pelvis comprises the hip bones, sacrum, and coccyx. Each hip bone is made up of three bones (ilium, ischium, and pubis). Each hip bone unites in front at the pubic symphysis, and joins the sacrum behind at the sacroiliac joint.

The male pelvis typically has a smaller heart-shaped inlet, a smaller pelvic outlet, and a more cone-shaped, longer cavity than the female pelvis. In addition, the male pelvis typically is distinguished by its larger bones, more defined muscle markings, and larger joint surfaces—reflecting the generally stronger build and heavier weight of men.

The function of the pelvis is to transfer weight from the vertebral column to the lower limbs, as well as to provide protection for the pelvic and lower abdominal organs.

On each side, the hip bone articulates with the head of the femur at the hip joint, and unites with the sacrum at the sacroiliac joint. The coccyx articulates with the sacrum at the sacrococcygeal joint.

anterior view

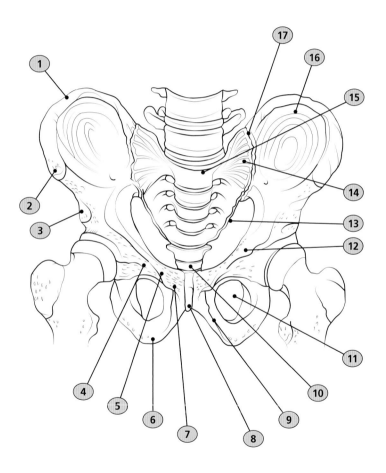

Bones of the Pelvis: Female

Key:

1 Sacroiliac joint
2 Anterior superior iliac spine
3 Iliopectineal eminence
4 Superior pubic ramus
5 Pubic tubercle
6 Pubic symphysis
7 Obturator foramen
8 Ischium
9 Coccyx
10 Pelvic sacral foramina
11 Iliac fossa
12 Iliac crest
13 Alar part of sacrum
14 Sacral promontory

Description:

The bony pelvis forms the skeletal framework for the pelvis.
It comprises the hip bones, sacrum, and coccyx. The two hip bones
are themselves made up of three fused bones (ilium, ischium, and
pubis), and each hip bone unites in front at the pubic symphysis and
joins the sacrum behind at the sacroiliac joint.

Generally, the female pelvis has a larger pelvic inlet and outlet
than the male pelvis. In addition, the length of the pelvic canal is
shorter in the female pelvis, and its walls are more parallel than those
of the male. The typical "gynecoid" pelvic inlet is wider than it is
deep, though the outlet is normally deeper than it is wide.

The bones that comprise the pelvis participate in a number of
articulations. The sacrum and coccyx articulate at the sacrococcygeal
joint. Each of the hip bones articulates with the femur at the hip joint—a
highly mobile ball-and-socket joint. The sacrum and the ilium of the
hip bone meet at the sacroiliac joint—this joint is synovial at the front
and fibrous at the back, and has only a small degree of movement.

anterior view

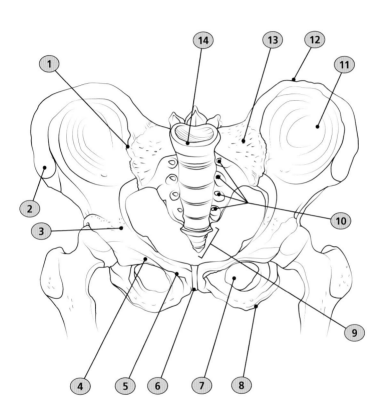

Bones of the Lower Limb

Key:
1 Femur
2 Patella
3 Tibia
4 Fibula
5 Talus
6 Tarsal bones
7 Metatarsal bones
8 Phalanges

Description:
The bones of the lower limb include the femur in the thigh, and the tibia and fibula in the leg. The femur is the longest bone in the body, and the tibia is the second longest. Body weight is transferred from the vertebral column to the hip bones and then to each femur.

The femur articulates with the hip bone at the top, and with the patella and tibia at its base. The tibia and fibula articulate with the talus (one of the tarsals) at the ankle joint.

anterior view—right limb

posterior view—left limb

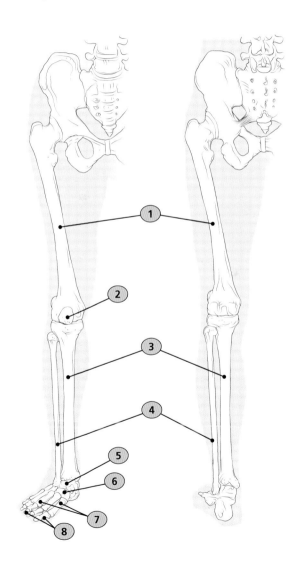

Femur

Key:

1 Greater trochanter
2 Head of femur
3 Fovea capitis
4 Neck of femur
5 Intertrochanteric ridge (crest)
6 Lesser trochanter
7 Linea aspera
8 Diaphysis
9 Popliteal surface
10 Lateral epicondyle
11 Medial epicondyle
12 Adductor tubercle
13 Medial condyle
14 Intercondylar fossa
15 Lateral condyle
16 Patellar surface

Description:

Extending from the hip to the knee, the femur (thigh bone) is the longest and strongest bone in the body. Features of the femur include a rounded head and a long neck with two enlargements—the greater trochanter and the lesser trochanter. These enlargements provide a point of attachment for the muscles of the upper leg. At the distal end of the femur are two protuberances—the lateral condyle and the medial condyle.

The head of the femur sits in a socket formed by the hip bones (ischium, ilium, and pubis). This ball-and-socket joint is extremely mobile. The distal end of the femur articulates with the tibia of the lower leg and the patella (kneecap) at the knee joint.

anterior view

posterior view

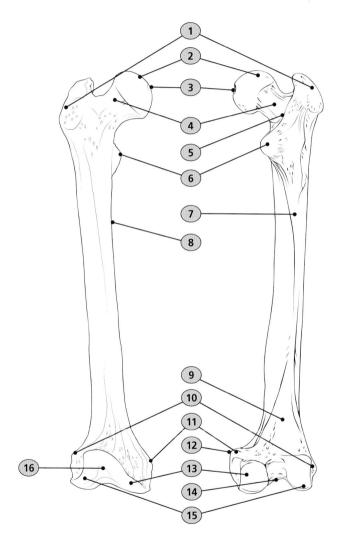

Tibia and Fibula

Key:

1	Lateral tibial condyle	**8**	Tibia
2	Intercondylar eminence	**9**	Fibula
3	Medial tibial condyle	**10**	Fibular notch
4	Head of fibula	**11**	Medial malleolus
5	Neck of fibula	**12**	Inferior articular surface
6	Tibial tuberosity	**13**	Lateral malleolus
7	Anterior border		

Description:

The tibia (commonly known as the shinbone) is the innermost bone of the leg and the thicker of the two bones. The second longest bone in the body, the tibia features a broad head and a cylindrical shaft that widens at the lower end to include the medial malleolus. The medial malleolus of the tibia is the small protruding bump on the inside of the ankle.

The fibula is the long slender bone on the outside of the leg, extending from just below the knee to the ankle, where its lower end forms the lateral side of the ankle joint.

anterior view

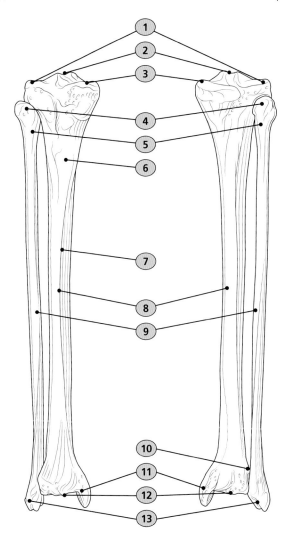

Bones of the Knee

Key:

1 Femoral shaft
2 Patella
3 Lateral condyle
4 Tibia
5 Fibula
6 Tibial plateau
7 Articular cartilage

Description:

The knee joint is a complex hinge joint between the femur, tibia, and patella. The lower end of the femur has a concave surface at the front, into which the back of the patella fits, and two rounded condyles at its base. The upper surface of the tibia is relatively flat. Depth to the tibial plateaus is provided by the medial and lateral menisci, which are wedge-shaped fibrocartilages. Each of the rounded condyles of the femur fits into the shallow sockets formed by the corresponding tibial plateau bounded by the menisci. The articulating surfaces are lined with hyaline cartilage.

lateral view—left limb

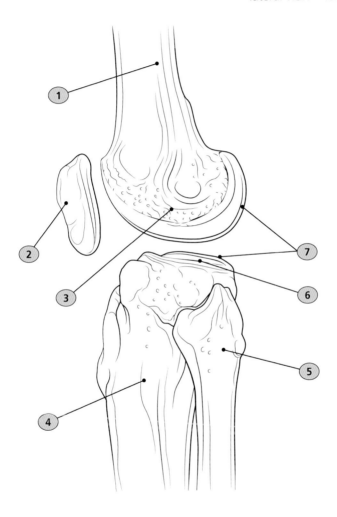

Bones of the Ankle and Foot

Key:

1 Fibula
2 Calcaneus
3 Cuboid
4 Metatarsal bones
5 Distal phalanges
6 Middle phalanges

7 Proximal phalanges
8 Cuneiform bones
9 Navicular
10 Talus
11 Tibia

Description:

The bones of the foot are the tarsals (seven bones in total—the talus, calcaneus, navicular, cuboid, and the three cuneiform bones [lateral, intermediate, and medial]); the five metatarsals; and the fourteen phalanges of the toes. The tarsus (the back half of the foot) is formed by the seven irregularly shaped tarsal bones. The foot is designed to support the body and to act as a lever to propel the body forward during walking. The segmented bone structure of the foot allows it to adapt to the shape of any surface, and enhances its propulsive effect during running.

   The segmented bone structure of the foot results in a large number of joints. At the back of the foot, the talus articulates with the tibia and fibula at the ankle joint. The tarsal bones are separated from one another by joints, which allow gliding movements to occur between them. The metatarsal bones form joints behind with the tarsus, and in front with the phalanges. Further joints occur between the proximal, middle, and distal phalanges.

lateral view—right limb

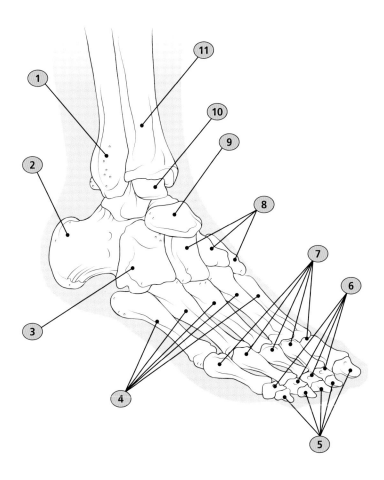

Skeletal System

Bones of the Ankle and Foot

Key:

1 Fibula
2 Cuboid
3 Distal phalanx
4 Proximal phalanx
5 First metatarsal
6 Cuneiform bones
7 Calcaneus
8 Navicular
9 Talus
10 Tibia

Description:
The ankle attaches the tibia and fibula of the leg to the talus
of the foot. Prominent features of the ankle joint include the medial
malleolus on the tibia and the lateral malleolus on the fibula. The two
malleoli, together with part of the tibia, form a socket in which the talus
can move.

The bones of the foot are the tarsals (seven bones in total—the
talus, calcaneus, navicular, cuboid, and the three cuneiform bones [lateral,
intermediate, and medial]); the five metatarsals; and the fourteen
phalanges of the toes. The tarsus (the back half of the foot) is formed by
the seven irregularly shaped tarsal bones.

medial view—right limb

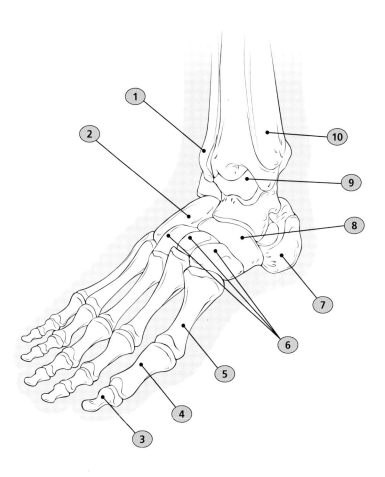

Joints (Articular System)

Wherever two bones meet, a joint is formed. Some are immobile, such as the fibrous gomphosis of the maxilla and mandible that anchor teeth in position, whereas others are highly mobile, such as the synovial ball and socket joints of the shoulder and hip. Some joints are immobile for most of one's life but can become mobile when required, such as the pubic symphysis and sacroiliac joints of the female pelvis that can become mobile to facilitate the birth of a child. Mobile synovial joints have joint surfaces covered by smooth hyaline cartilage and separated by a thin lubricating film of synovial fluid.

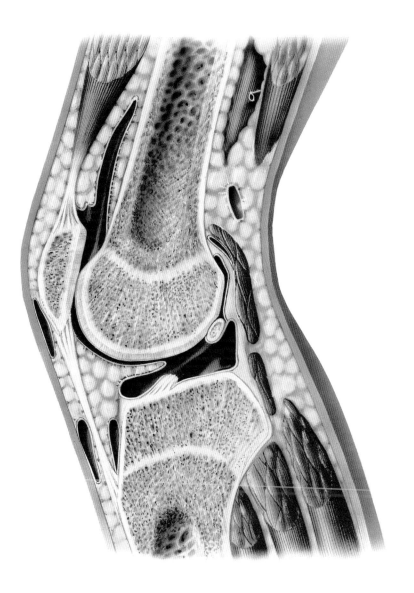

Articulations

Key:

1 Carpal bones

2 Radius

3 Ulna

4 Head of femur (ball)

5 Acetabular fossa (socket)

6 Scaphoid bone

7 Radius

8 Ulna

Description:

A joint is where two bones meet and articulate. The bones may be separated by cartilage and often fluid. Not all joints are mobile—there is no perceptible movement at the sutures of the skull, and only limited movement occurs in joints such as the pubic symphysis. The most mobile joints are the synovial joints. Smooth cartilage covers the articular surfaces, which are enclosed in a membrane-lined capsule. The synovial membrane releases synovial fluid, which lubricates the joint and reduces friction. Synovial joint types include gliding (plane), ball-and-socket, ellipsoidal (condyloid), saddle, hinge, and pivot.

A gliding joint allows only slight sliding movement (e.g., between the carpal bones of the wrist). The ball-and-socket joint is the most mobile joint type in the body. The rounded head of a bone unites with a socket cavity in another bone. Examples of ball-and-socket joints include the shoulder joint and the hip joint. Ellipsoidal joints allow movement in two directions, such as that between the distal surfaces of the forearm bones (radius and ulna) and the adjacent carpal bones.

Continued on page 118

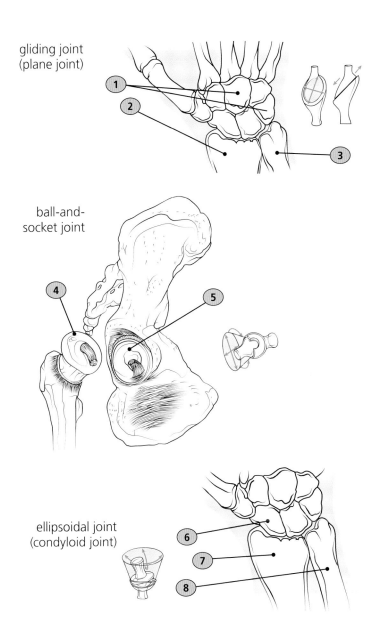

gliding joint (plane joint)

1
2
3

ball-and-socket joint

4
5

ellipsoidal joint (condyloid joint)

6
7
8

Joints

Articulations

Key:

1 Metacarpal bone of thumb
2 Trapezium bone
3 Humerus
4 Coronoid process of ulna
5 Trochlea (of humerus)
6 Olecranon
7 Ulna
8 Radius
9 Atlas
10 Axis

Description:

Continued from page 116

The saddle joint is a highly mobile joint that allows sliding movement in two directions—this type of joint is found where the metacarpal of the thumb meets the trapezium of the carpus (wrist). A hinge joint can move in one plane only, providing flexion and extension. The elbow is an example of a hinge joint. The knee joint, however, is more complex than the elbow, allowing some rotation around the long axis of the tibia, and is more properly called a bicondylar joint. A pivot joint allows rotational movement around a single axis—as found between the atlas (C1) and axis (C2) of the vertebral column.

saddle joint

hinge joint

pivot joint

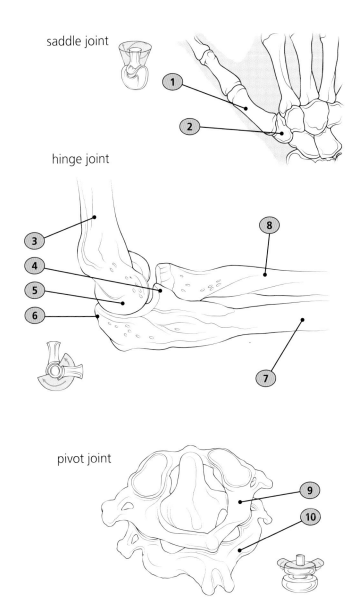

Joints

Shoulder Joint

Key:

1 Clavicle
2 Coracoid process
3 Acromion
4 Head of humerus
5 Glenoid cavity
6 Humerus

Description:

The humerus of the arm and the scapula are the two major components of the shoulder joint, with the clavicle providing stability. The clavicle and scapula form the pectoral girdle.

The lateral angle of the scapula is flattened to form a shallow cavity in which the head of the humerus sits, forming the shoulder (glenohumeral) joint—a ball-and-socket joint allowing movement of the arm to occur in almost any direction. The socket, which is formed by the glenoid cavity of the scapula, is very shallow and has a small contact area, relative to the head of the humerus, which forms the ball. Only a small part of the head of the humerus is in contact with the glenoid cavity at any time, making the joint extremely mobile, but also making it relatively unstable. A ring of fibrocartilage, the glenoid labrum, which encircles the edge of the glenoid cavity, deepens the socket slightly and increases the contact area. The joint surfaces are covered by smooth glassy cartilage, and a relatively loose capsule holds the two bones together. The capsule is lined with synovial membrane, which releases synovial fluid to lubricate the cartilage surface and reduce friction. The shoulder joint is bridged and protected above by the coracoacromial arch, formed by the acromion behind, the coracoid process in front, and the coracoacromial ligament passing between them.

anterior view

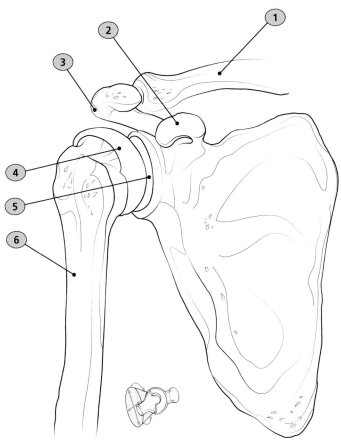

movement of
the shoulder
(glenohumeral joint)

Joints

Ligaments of the Shoulder

Key:

1 Acromioclavicular ligament
2 Acromion
3 Coracoacromial ligament
4 Coracohumeral ligament
5 Transverse humeral ligament

6 Humerus
7 Glenohumeral ligaments
8 Scapula
9 Coracoid process
10 Clavicle
11 Coracoclavicular ligament

Description:

The ball-and-socket joint of the shoulder is an extremely mobile joint. Its great flexibility and range of movement is made possible by the round ball of the humerus and the shallow surface of the glenoid cavity of the scapula. A number of strong ligaments keep the shoulder joint stable, including the glenohumeral ligaments, which link the humerus and scapula, and the coracohumeral ligament, which links the humerus and the coracoid process.

Adding extra stability to the region are the coracoacromial ligament, which joins the coracoid process and the acromion; the acromioclavicular ligament, which joins the acromion to the clavicle; and the coracoclavicular ligament, which joins the coracoid process and the clavicle. The transverse humeral ligament spans the sulcus between the two tubercles at the head of the humerus, acting to hold down the tendons of the biceps brachii muscle.

anterior view

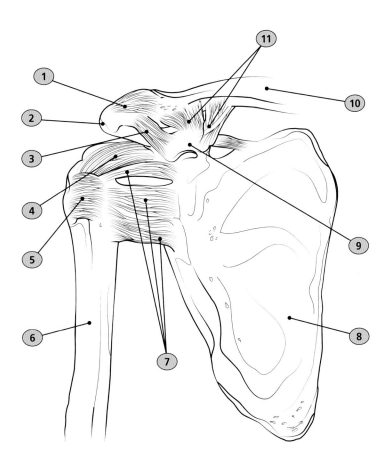

Joints

Elbow Joint

Key:
1. Humerus
2. Coronoid process of ulna
3. Head of radius
4. Neck of radius
5. Shaft of radius
6. Shaft of ulna
7. Olecranon
8. Trochlea of humerus
9. Medial epicondyle of humerus

Description:

The elbow is the joint between the expanded distal end of the humerus of the arm, and the proximal ends of the ulna and radius of the forearm. The radius is on the thumb side of the arm, and the ulna is on the side of the little finger.

   The proximal end of the ulna articulates with the distal end of the humerus—this articulation forms a hinge joint, allowing flexion (bending) and extension (straightening). The articulation between the radius and ulna forms a pivot joint, which allows rotational movement of the radius around the ulna.

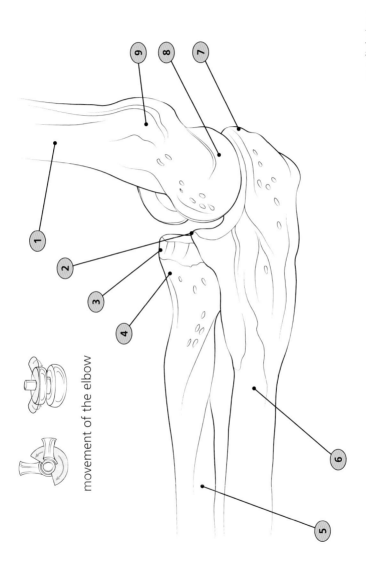

medial view

movement of the elbow

Ligaments of the Elbow

Key:

1 Shaft of radius
2 Oblique cord
3 Ulna
4 Annular ligament of radius
5 Ulnar collateral ligament
6 Olecranon
7 Humerus

Description:

The bones of the elbow joint—humerus, radius, and ulna—are held together by strong fibrous ligaments. Joining the humerus to the ulna and olecranon, on the medial (inner) side of the joint, is the ulnar collateral ligament. On the lateral side of the joint, the radial collateral ligament joins the humerus to the radius, affixing to the radius at the annular ligament, which joins the head of the radius to the ulna.

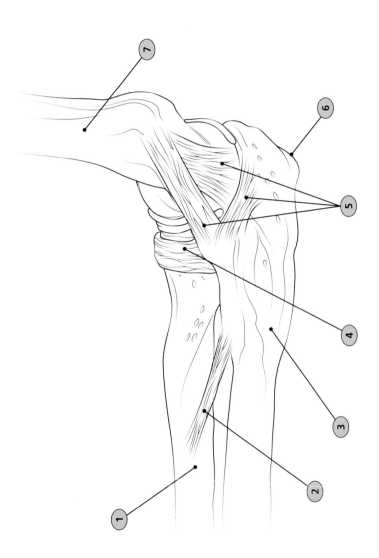

medial view

Ligaments of the Wrist and Hand

Key:

1 Palmar ligaments and articular capsule of interphalangeal joints
2 Proximal phalanges
3 Palmar metacarpal ligaments
4 Pisometacarpal ligament
5 Pisohamate ligament
6 Capitotriquetral ligament
7 Ulnar collateral ligament
8 Palmar radioulnar ligament
9 Ulna
10 Radius
11 Ulnolunate part (palmar ulnocarpal ligaments)
12 Radioscapholunate part (palmar radiocarpal ligaments)
13 Radiocapitate part (palmar radiocarpal ligaments)
14 Trapezium
15 Palmar carpometacarpal ligaments
16 Collateral digital ligaments
17 Metacarpal bones
18 Metacarpophalangeal ligaments
19 Distal phalanx of thumb
20 Middle phalanges
21 Distal phalanges

Description:

The joints of the wrist are enclosed by a fibrous joint capsule and bound together by many ligaments. The radial and ulnar collateral ligaments are rounded cords that attach the radius and ulnar to proximal (upper) carpal bones. There are also broad ligaments attaching the radius to proximal carpal bones—the palmar (or anterior) radiocarpal ligament (on the palm of the hand) and the dorsal (or posterior) radiocarpal ligament (on the back of the hand). The transverse carpal ligament (also called the flexor retinaculum) spans the carpal bones, and inside the joint capsule the intercarpal ligaments (dorsal and palmar) connect the individual carpal bones. The carpometacarpal ligaments (dorsal and palmar) join the distal (lower) carpal bones to the bases of the metacarpal bones of the hand.

palmar view—right limb

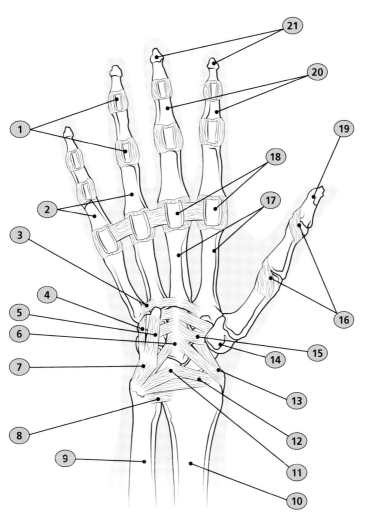

Hip Joint

Key:

1 Acetabular rim
2 Head of femur
3 Neck of femur
4 Ischium
5 Greater trochanter
6 Femur
7 Ilium

Description:

The hip (coxal or innominate) bone is made up of three bones—the ilium, ischium, and pubis. The three bones fuse with each other at the acetabulum at 14–16 years of age. The crest of the ilium is located at the waist, laterally, below the ribs. The two ischia feature tuberosities at their base. The pubic bones are at the front of the hip bone. The left and right hip bones and the sacrum form the bony pelvis. The hip joint is formed by the acetabulum—a cup-shaped socket—and the rounded head of the femur. The hip transmits the entire weight of the upper body to the head and neck of each femur.

The hip is a ball-and-socket joint formed at the point where the femur meets the acetabulum of the hip bone. The joint is enclosed in a fibrous capsule that is loose enough to permit free movement, yet strong enough to hold the femoral head in place. More than half of the rounded head of the femur is held within the acetabulum and surrounding cartilage, making the joint stable and strong, with capability of rotation second only to the shoulder joint and limited only by the flexibility of its supporting ligaments (iliofemoral, ischiofemoral, and pubofemoral).

anterior view—left limb

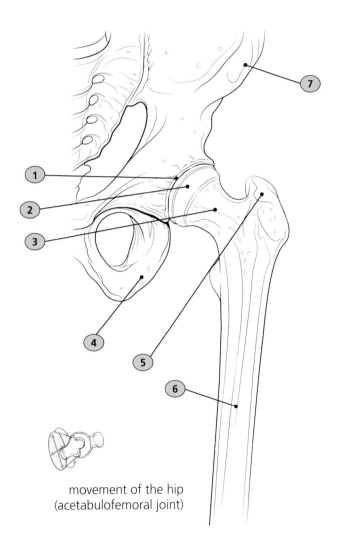

movement of the hip
(acetabulofemoral joint)

Ligaments of the Pelvis and Hip

Key:

1 Iliac crest
2 Sacrotuberous and sacrospinous ligaments
3 Ventral sacrococcygeal ligament
4 Pubic symphysis
5 Pubofemoral ligament
6 Iliofemoral ligament
7 Anterior sacroiliac ligament
8 Iliolumbar ligament
9 Anterior longitudinal ligament

Description:

There are many ligaments in the pelvis, which connect and strengthen the articulations between the sacrum, coccyx, ilium, and pubic bones. Connecting the tuberosities of the sacrum and the ilium is the interosseous sacroiliac ligament. Also between the sacrum and ilium are the anterior sacroiliac ligament and the two posterior sacroiliac ligaments—short (upper) and long (lower). Between the sacrum and coccyx are the sacrococcygeal ligaments (anterior, posterior, and lateral). Between the sacrum and ischium are the sacrotuberous ligament, which connects the ischial tuberosity of the ischium to the sacrum and coccyx; and the sacrospinous ligament, which connects the ischial spine to the sacrum and coccyx. There is also the iliolumbar ligament, which connects the iliac crest to the L4 and L5 vertebrae. Connecting the two pubic bones are the anterior, posterior, superior, and arcuate ligaments.

anterior view

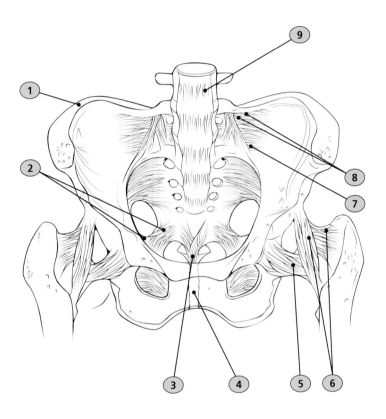

Joints

Knee Joint

Key:

1 Femur
2 Articular cartilage
3 Patella
4 Lateral condyle
5 Tibial plateau
6 Fibula
7 Tibia

Description:

The knee joint is a complex bicondylar joint formed by the femur, tibia, and patella, and because its adjacent surfaces do not fit tightly together, it relies mainly on ligaments, menisci, and muscles for stability. The three bones of the knee joint are united by a fibrous capsule that encloses a single large joint cavity between the bones.

The inside of the capsule is lined with synovial membrane, which releases synovial fluid to lubricate the joint surfaces to keep them friction-free. Pouches of synovial membrane extend beyond the confines of the joint capsule forming sacs known as bursae, and making the knee joint the most extensive of any joint in the body. The knee's main movements are flexion and extension, although some backward and forward gliding movement and some rotation also occur.

lateral view—left limb

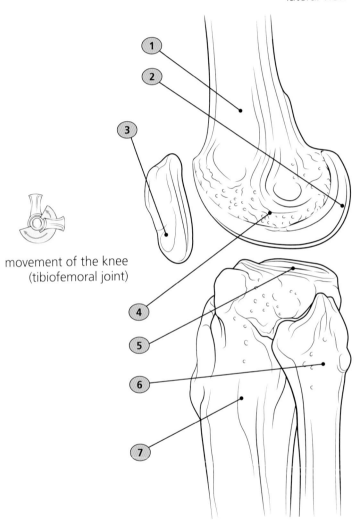

movement of the knee
(tibiofemoral joint)

Bones and Ligaments of the Knee

Key:

1 Femur
2 Posterior cruciate ligament
3 Lateral condyle of femur
4 Fibular (lateral) collateral ligament
5 Lateral meniscus
6 Anterior cruciate ligament
7 Patella (reflected)
8 Tibia
9 Patellar ligament
10 Tibial (medial) collateral ligament
11 Medial meniscus
12 Medial condyle of femur

Description:

The knee joint is formed by the femur, patella, and tibia. The lower end of the femur has a concave surface at the front, into which the back of the patella fits, and two rounded condyles at its base. Depth to the tibial plateaus is provided by the medial and lateral menisci. Each of the rounded condyles of the femur fits into the shallow sockets formed by the corresponding tibial plateau and menisci.

Ligaments strengthen the knee joint and limit excessive movements. The medial side is reinforced by the tibial (medial) collateral ligament, which extends from the sides of the femoral condyle down onto the shaft of the tibia. The lateral side is reinforced by the fibular (lateral) collateral ligament, which extends from the lateral femoral condyle down to the head of the fibula. Inside the joint capsule are the two cruciate ligaments, which prevent excessive forward or backward gliding during flexion and extension of the knee.

anterior view—right limb

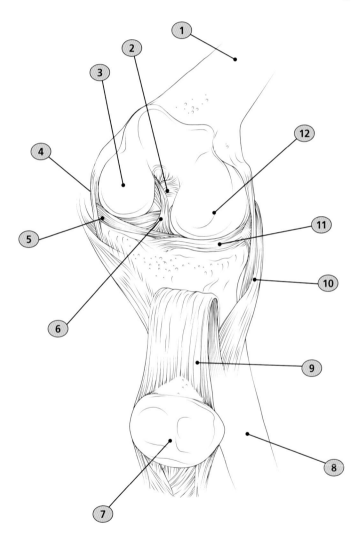

Joints

Bones and Ligaments of the Ankle

Key:

1 Tibia
2 Medial malleolus
3 Deltoid (medial) ligament
4 Posterior talocalcaneal ligament
5 Calcaneus
6 Talus
7 Calcaneofibular ligament
8 Posterior talofibular ligament
9 Lateral malleolus
10 Posterior tibiofibular ligament
11 Fibula
12 Interosseous membrane

Description:

The ankle attaches the tibia and fibula of the leg to the talus—one of the bones of the ankle. Prominent features of the ankle joint include the medial malleolus, a bony protrusion on the end of the tibia, and the lateral malleolus, a similar bony landmark at the end of the fibula. The two malleoli, together with a part of the tibia, form a socket in which the talus can move. Several ligaments make the ankle joint strong and stable. On the medial side of the joint, the broad, strong, triangular deltoid (medial) ligament connects the medial malleolus of the tibia to three of the tarsal bones (talus, navicular, and calcaneus). On the lateral side of the joint, three cordlike ligaments—the anterior talofibular ligament, the posterior talofibular ligament, and the calcaneofibular ligament—attach the lateral malleolus of the fibula to the talus and calcaneus.

   The ankle joint—formed by the tibia, fibula, and talus—is a synovial hinge joint and is fairly stable. The joint formed by these three bones allows the heel to be raised from the ground, as in pointing one's toes (plantarflexion), and for the upper surface of the foot to be brought closer to the front of the leg (dorsiflexion).

posterior view—right limb

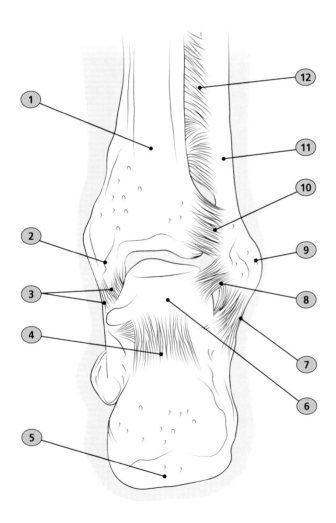

Joints

Ligaments of the Ankle and Foot

Key:

1 Fibula
2 Anterior tibiofibular ligament
3 Posterior tibiofibular ligament
4 Calcaneofibular ligament
5 Calcaneus
6 Talocalcaneal ligaments
7 Bifurcate ligament
8 Dorsal calcaneocuboid ligament
9 Dorsal cuneocuboid ligament
10 Dorsal metatarsal ligaments
11 Dorsal tarsometatarsal ligaments
12 Dorsal intercuneiform ligament
13 Dorsal cuneonavicular ligaments
14 Dorsal cuboideonavicular ligament
15 Anterior talofibular ligament
16 Tibia

Description:
The principal ligaments involved in strengthening the ankle joint are the deltoid (medial) ligament on the medial (inner) side of the joint, and the three lateral ligaments—the anterior talofibular ligament, the posterior talofibular ligament, and the calcaneofibular ligament—on the outer side of the joint. Ligaments strengthen the joints between each of the bones of the talus, while small ligaments attach the talus bones to adjoining metatarsal bones.

lateral view—right limb

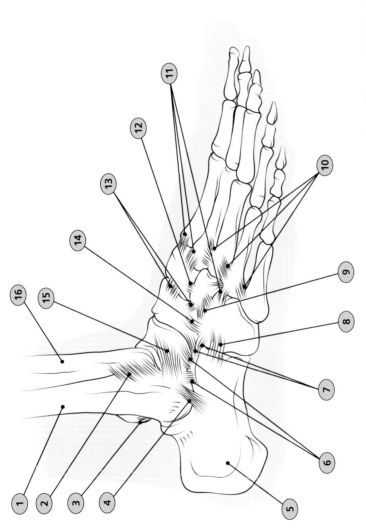

Index

Index